Non-Prescription Drugs
and Their Side Effects

Robert J. Benowicz

GROSSET & DUNLAP
A FILMWAYS COMPANY
Publishers · New York

Copyright © 1977 by Robert J. Benowicz
All rights reserved
Published simultaneously in Canada
Library of Congress catalog card number: 77-71741
ISBN   0-448-14323-2 (hardcover edition)
ISBN   0-448-14324-0 (paperback edition)
Printed in the United States of America

CONTENTS

Introduction

Why a book about non-prescription drugs? After all, each of us is free to purchase and use these over-the-counter products just as freely as we buy and consume candy or chewing gum. There are no laws which prohibit the sale of these medications. They are available not only from drugstores but from supermarkets, discount houses, and even newsstands. Can such products be anything but safe, effective, and a benefit to all?

Although not a physician, a pharmacist, or a medical professional, I am a friend, a consumer, and a biochemist. Recent personal experiences have made me aware of how little is known, even among professional scientists, about the hazards involved in the casual consumption of non-prescription medications. Within one month three close friends were rushed to the hospital, suffering because of the unwitting misuse of over-the-counter drugs.

One friend, a brilliant research biologist, fell asleep at the wheel of her car. She had taken her regular non-prescription medication for hay fever and forgot or was unaware that antihistamines often induce drowsiness or sleep. Another friend, a foreign correspondent, suffered from a minor bacterial infection which his physician treated with an antibiotic (tetracycline). Not until his infection became life-threatening did this very intelligent man tell his doctor that the antibiotic upset his stomach. With each dose of antibiotic he was taking a concentrated non-prescription antacid. Since antacids dramatically reduce the effectiveness of tetracycline, his infection went largely unchecked. A third friend, a high-powered executive secretary, was taken to the hospital with severely bleeding ulcers. Her condition had become acute because she regularly used 2–4 aspirin a day to relieve the tension produced by her job. Fortunately, all three of these close friends and colleagues regained their health, but not without considerable pain, suffering, and expense. Although their experiences are not typical of the vast majority of us who use non-prescription medications, they are by no means unique.

How can such harrowing experiences be avoided? If we turned to medical doctors for every headache, sniffle, or sneeze, the American health care system would collapse. Intelligent self-treatment and self-medication have always had and probably will continue to have a major role in health care. But when faced with minor illness, how do we sensibly select or evaluate an appropriate product without risking serious complications?

Our highly technological and capitalistic society has managed to formulate, fabricate, market, and promote hundreds of thousands of different non-prescription medications. On entering the modern drugstore we may be confronted with as many as 200 different brand-name products for the relief of cold symptoms. Each one is apt to be cleverly packaged and displayed without revealing very much about its real potential for good or evil. Many labels tell almost nothing about a drug's rational uses, its concentrations of medically active ingredients, or the potential for negative side effects and adverse reactions. Many labels which do provide such information require a high-powered magnifying glass for legibility and a medical dictionary for comprehension. Faced by such a dazzling and puzzling array, the chances of making a rational choice seem slim indeed. Nevertheless, there are many steps that we can follow in finding the non-prescription medication with a maximum potential for relief and a minimum potential for negative side effects and adverse reactions. Given adequate information, rational choices can be made.

Sources of Information: The Coming Revolution in Non-Prescription, Over-the-Counter (OTC) Medications

In May of 1972 the Food and Drug Administration began an exhaustive evaluation of all non-prescription medications. Its purpose is to establish rigorous standards for the safety, effectiveness, and labeling of over-the-counter products. Its appraisal is based on the work of independent advisory review panels that judge all medically active ingredients in specific classes of non-prescription products, e.g., internal analgesics (aspirin), antacids, laxatives, etc. Manufacturers of over-the-counter medications have been invited to submit fundamental information about their products to the FDA. This information is now a matter of public record. Preliminary recommendations concerning safety, effectiveness, and labeling are periodically submitted to the commissioner of the FDA and are published in the *Federal Register*. It is these advisory panel reports plus the manufacturer's product submissions which form much of the basis for this book. Although the entire review of non-prescription medications will not be completed before the mid-1980s, the preliminary findings probably represent the most comprehensive and reliable assessment of over-the-counter products available.

The American Pharmaceutical Association publishes a *Handbook of Nonprescription Drugs.* The fifth edition of January, 1977, is a superb and comprehensive guide to more than 1500 OTC products and the conditions they are intended to relieve. Its language is technical and appropriate to the pharmacists for whom it was written. Much of the information used here has been checked against that included in the *Handbook.* Many of the questions you will ask yourself as you use this book are correlated with those the *Handbook* advises a pharmacist to ask his clients before recommending a specific product. Your awareness will assist in his or her selection of a product appropriate for you.

Because the simultaneous use of prescription and non-prescription drugs can produce serious side effects and adverse reactions, most chapters contain a list of prescription medications which should not be used with specific non-prescription medications unless your doctor approves. Edward L. Stern's *Prescription Drugs and Their Side Effects,* also published by Grosset & Dunlap, is an excellent layman's reference to such medications.

More technical materials have been drawn from the 1977 *Physicians' Desk Reference, Hazards of Medication* by Eric W. Martin, and *Evaluations of Drug Interactions* published by the American Pharmaceutical Association. The scientific language typical of medical texts has been simplified here. However, some technical terms remain. Don't be intimidated by them. The labels of many reputable products include them, and they are your key to understanding the contents. Feel no embarrassment about writing them down and taking them with you to a drugstore.

How to Use This Book

Non-Prescription Drugs and Their Side Effects is not intended to promote or to discredit any over-the-counter product. It is intended to assist you in understanding the appropriate use and the potential for misuse of non-prescription medications.

Self-medication with over-the-counter (OTC) drugs is generally reasonable for the relief of symptoms produced by minor and self-limiting (temporary) diseases that do not require medical supervision. The major classes of such conditions provide basic chapter divisions for this book. Each chapter is further subdivided into 3 sections.[1]

---

1. Products which are not generally thought of as specific for a particular disease, e.g., vitamins, soaps, certain skin preparations, etc., will be considered in later volumes in this series.

1. **General Considerations** This section provides basic information about a disorder, its suitability for self-treatment, more serious disease conditions which may mimic its symptoms, forms of non-drug therapies, and the kinds of active ingredients frequently included in non-prescription products.

2. **Self-Treatment** This section (indicated by gray tint) can help you quickly determine whether self-medication is appropriate for your symptoms. It lists those conditions for which self-medication *may* be appropriate, when self-medication is probably *not* advisable, a series of questions to ask yourself before choosing a product, and a listing of the medically active ingredients frequently included in brand-name products.

3. **Product Charts** This section lists a representative sampling of generally available non-prescription products. It includes brand name, manufacturer, delivery form (tablet, powder, capsule, etc.), and their concentrations of active ingredients in the usual dosage strengths. If you do not find an entry for a given product, comparison of the label with listed products will help you evaluate the brand in question. The alphabetical index at the end of the book gives you an immediate reference to the brand name medications included in the product charts.

Some General Principles of Self-Medication

Rely on your registered pharmacist for advice and assistance. It is generally agreed that the average American pharmacist is as well acquainted with non-prescription medications and their possible interactions with other drugs as the average physician. Follow your pharmacist's advice. It is professional, and it is free.

Don't hesitate to consult your doctor at any time. If you have any uncertainty about the selection or evaluation of a non-prescription product, he or she will probably be happy to recommend one most appropriate for you without charge.

If you have any question or concern about any form of self-treatment or self-medication with non-prescription drugs, seeking your doctor's advice cannot be too strongly recommended. Always get his or her advice if—

- you are taking any prescription medication.
- you suffer from any chronic, acute, or debilitating disease.
- you are pregnant or nursing a baby.
- you or the person for whom you are responsible is either very young or very old.
- any symptoms become severe and/or chronic.

Avoid the use of combination products, e.g., those containing more than two medically active ingredients. Single ingredient medications are the most desirable since they reduce the possibility of poisoning, allergic reactions, and negative side effects.

Avoid the purchase of any product that doesn't list ingredients by name and by concentration.

Keep all medications out of the reach of children.

Non-Prescription Drugs and Their Side Effects was written for you. Your family. Your friends. It was written for you to use. To help you understand the appropriate use and potential for misuse of over-the-counter medications. To help you make intelligent decisions about self-treatment and self-medication. It is not intended as an encyclopedic listing of all non-prescription products. It is not a medical or a pharmacological text nor the last word in drug information. Every individual is different, and drugs affect people in different ways. It is, however, designed to be an easy-to-follow, basic reference source for consumers written in easy-to-understand language.

1
PAIN
FEVER
INFLAMMATION

GENERAL CONSIDERATIONS

Aspirin and Other Salicylates

Aspirin[1] is probably the most used and abused of non-prescription drugs. Its medically active ingredient forms when aspirin or a related salicylate compound[2] dissolves in water. The resulting solution can relieve certain kinds of pain, reduce fever, and ease some forms of joint inflammation.

Pain-reducing, or analgesic, effects are most often noted with headaches from sinus pressure or simple tension, the muscular soreness (*myalgia*) of menstrual cramping or muscle strain, the nerve pain (*neuralgia*) of minor toothache, and the joint soreness (*arthralgia*) of arthritis or bursitis.

Fever-reducing, or antipyretic effects of the salicylates result from increased dispersion of body heat, which does not interfere with your body's defenses. Because fever usually comes with potentially serious infections, be cautious about treating yourself with aspirin or an aspirin substitute. Treating a low-grade fever arising from the flu or a common cold is reasonable. Treating a fever arising from uncertain origins is *not* reasonable, and your doctor should be consulted.

Anti-inflammatory activity of the salicylates reduces the joint inflammation of arthritis or bursitis. Although the relief is undeniable, effective dosages exceed those recommended for self-medication, and prudent treatment requires your doctor's supervision.

Possible Side Effects and Drug Interactions   Although aspirin and aspirin substitutes are useful in treating mild to moderate pain and/or

---

1. Acetylsalicylic acid
2. Sodium salicylate, choline salicylate, salicylsalicylic acid, or calcium carbaspirin

fever, widespread advertisement, availability, and public acceptance obscure the dangers of uncritical use.

Alcohol Both alcohol and salicylates irritate the lining of your digestive tract. Taken together, they may cause stomach upset and internal bleeding. Don't use aspirin to treat a "hangover."

Allergy Sensitivity to salicylates—particularly to aspirin—can cause you severe breathing difficulty, skin rashes, and/or shock. Although this reaction is typical of fewer than 1% of the general population, its frequency approaches 5% among those with a history of asthma.

Blood-clotting and anticoagulant medications Because salicylates interfere with normal blood clotting and promote internal bleeding, their use in combination with prescribed anticoagulants magnifies the effects of the prescribed drugs and may cause severe bleeding.

Diabetes Salicylates increase the effect of oral hypoglycemics (insulin-like drugs). When taken together, blood sugar levels are depressed more than intended, and insulin shock may result.

Gout and other kidney diseases Aspirin and other salicylates interfere with drugs intended for the treatment of gout and other kidney disorders. Although the exact reason is not known, frequent use can damage kidney tissue.

Misdiagnosis Since aspirin and other analgesics relieve symptomatic pain, such relief may mask serious medical problems. This masking effect is particularly common with chest or abdominal pain that has not come from a known injury or strain. Masked symptoms may indicate disease of the stomach, heart, gall bladder, or appendix.

Overdose Poisoning results from overdose and you may recognize it by a ringing sensation in the ears, nausea, impaired vision, mental confusion, digestive disturbance, and/or rashes. It can be fatal and is the primary cause of death by poisoning among children under 5.

Stomach upset Each week an estimated 30 million Americans take aspirin or related products to relieve their headaches. Of these an estimated 1 in 20, or 1.5 million, suffer some form of indigestion, nausea or vomiting. Although these side effects may be eased by buffered products or by drinking a buffering liquid such as milk with unbuffered products, the use of salicylates if you have a peptic ulcer or other digestive ailment can cause severe irritation, damage or bleeding along your digestive tract.

Dosage The Food and Drug Administration (FDA) recommends that you do not take more than 4 grams of salicylate, equally distributed at 4- to 6-hour intervals, over any 24-hour period. Effective single dosages fall between a recommended minimum of 325 milligrams (5 grains) and a maximum of 650 milligrams (10 grains). You should not take aspirin or other salicylate for more than a week to 10 days without your doctor's supervision and should stop at the first signs of any side effect or adverse reaction.

Children's dosages   Be certain to follow the manufacturer's recommendations with the greatest care. If the label on your product has no information about children's dosages, use a brand that does.

Alternatives to Aspirin and Related Salicylates

Salicylamide   A compound inferior to the salicylates in pain- and fever-reducing effectiveness, its attractions are the speed with which it enters the bloodstream and the comparative rarity of allergic reactions. Although blood-clotting mechanisms and oral anticoagulants are apparently unaffected by the compound, salicylamide can have the same negative side effects and adverse reactions as the salicylates. It most often comes in combination with aspirin and/or its alternatives to promote an initial, rapid relief from pain or fever. Its total effectiveness in combination has yet to be determined, but it is *less* potent than equal doses of aspirin or other aspirin substitutes.

p-Aminophenols: Acetaminophen and Phenacetin   These 2 compounds are roughly equal in pain- and fever-reducing activity to aspirin, but have no significant anti-inflammatory effect. You can use them to treat the same kinds of headache, myalgia, neuralgia, and fever as the salicylates. Inside your body the majority of a phenacetin dosage is converted into acetaminophen.

Possible Side Effects and Drug Interactions of p-Aminophenols   Because acetaminophen and phenacetin produce fewer side effects than the salicylates—notably fewer allergic reactions, little interference with diabetic or kidney medications, and little incidence of digestive disturbance—both compounds have gained increased favor among doctors, pharmacists, and the general public. However, neither is free from potentially negative effects.

Blood clotting   Although neither acetaminophen nor phenacetin alone tends to cause bleeding in the digestive tract, acetaminophen can increase the action of oral anticoagulants and produce internal bleeding.

The repeated use of phenacetin can activate certain kinds of anemia. The effect is particularly dangerous if you suffer from an inherited disease known as glucose-6-dehydrogenase (G-6-D) deficiency. Although rare among Americans of Western European origin, its incidence is as high as 15% among American Blacks. If you have inherited the disorder and regularly take phenacetin, you run a high risk of serious anemia.

Misdiagnosis   As with the salicylates, medication with aminophenols may mask symptoms of serious disease.

Overdose   Because of a growing tendency to substitute aminophenols for aspirin, increased incidences of aminophenol poisoning are occurring. Be aware that symptoms of overdose include nausea, vomiting, and loss of appetite.

Dosage   Single doses of between 325 mg (5 gr) and 650 mg (10 gr) at 4- to 6-hour intervals are generally recommended for self-treatment. Maximum daily consumption should not exceed 2.6 g (40 gr), which is considerably less than the 4 g (61.5 gr) maximum for aspirin. Where manufacturers advise lower individual or total daily amounts, take their advice.
Children's dosages   Be sure to follow the manufacturer's recommendations with the greatest care. If the label has no information about children, use a brand that does.

Combination Products

A majority of non-prescription pain- and fever-reducers offer some combination of aspirin, other salicylates, salicylamide, acetaminophen, and/or phenacetin. There is little evidence that the effects of such combinations are more than simply additive. A product that contains 325 mg (5 gr) of aspirin and 325 mg (5 gr) of acetaminophen is probably no more effective than alternatives containing 650 mg (10 gr) of either aspirin or acetaminophen alone.

Because salicylamide is less potent than either the salicylates or aminophenols, its inclusion in a combination means the product is less effective than equal doses of any other combination of aspirin and/or aspirin substitute.

Possible Side Effects and Drug Interactions   Combination analgesics containing fractions of aspirin, the other salicylates, salicylamide, and/or aminophenols confront you with the hazards typical of each. A product containing portions of aspirin and acetaminophen is apt to produce the side effects of *both* the salicylates and the aminophenols. In some cases—notably the combination of aspirin, phenacetin, and caffeine (APC)—you may suffer side effects that would not occur if you took either medically active ingredient alone. The mixture of aspirin with phenacetin can produce serious kidney damage, starting with digestive upset or blood in the urine.

Dosage   Follow the manufacturer's advice about individual dosage, spacing of doses, and maximum daily dosage.
Children's dosages   The use of combination products is probably unwise unless otherwise directed by your pediatrician.

Additives to Aspirin and Aspirin Substitutes

Buffers Because acetylsalicylic acid can irritate the lining of your digestive tract, buffering compounds[1] are frequently added to aspirin to combat stomach upset. These compounds reduce internal bleeding, dissolve more rapidly, and enter your bloodstream faster than non-buffered aspirin. However, there is no certain proof that relief is any quicker with buffered than with non-buffered forms. Evidence does exist that a full glass of milk or water taken with non-buffered aspirin provides the same protection as the buffering agents.

Caffeine The addition of small amounts of caffeine is common among pain- and fever-reducing products. It stimulates your circulation and may distribute the pain-reliever more rapidly. However, there is no convincing evidence that caffeine accelerates or improves the effectiveness of either the salicylates or aminophenols. The amount present in non-prescription analgesics is generally less than that in half a cup of coffee.

Antihistamines A number of products contain antihistamines.[2] In theory they minimize some allergic reactions, relax muscles associated with tension-induced pain, and/or promote sleep at night. Evidence for these claims is inconclusive.

Delivery Forms

Tablet The most common. Intended to dissolve completely on contact with the watery medium of the stomach and small intestine before absorption into your bloodstream.

Timed-release Either capsules or tablets that dissolve at different rates in digestive fluids over long periods of time. These are not meant for rapid relief but for extended activity, generally at bedtime.

Effervescing powders or tablets These are dissolved in water before ingestion and are more readily absorbed than standard tablets or capsules. They are usually buffered to prevent stomach upset. Because they contain high concentrations of sodium or potassium, avoid them if you are on a salt-restricted diet.

Coated capsules The medically active ingredient is surrounded by a coating to prevent its dissolving before reaching the small intestine. This avoids possible irritation of the stomach lining. Complete break-

---

1. Such as aluminum and magnesium hydroxide, aluminum and magnesium carbonate, sodium bicarbonate, etc.
2. In the form of methapyrilene or phenyltoloxamine

down of the protective coating and the release of the active ingredient(s) in the small intestine can be highly erratic.

Liquid Predissolved salicylates are most rapidly absorbed and minimize the risks of stomach upset. They are usually contained in a solution which also includes artificial flavoring and some alcohol.

SELF-TREATMENT

The Use of Aspirin, Other Salicylates, Salicylamide, or Aminophenols May Be Indicated If You Wish to Relieve the Symptoms of—

- sinus or tension headache.
- muscular ache, pain, or soreness resulting from menstrual cramping, minor injury, or strain.
- neuralgia.
- mild to moderate fever (up to 100° F.) associated with the common cold or the flu.
- combinations of the above typical of the common cold or the flu.

Before beginning self-treatment, be sure to review the precautions against the use of aspirin or other salicylates listed below.

Don't Treat Yourself with Aspirin, Other Salicylates, or Salicylamide if—

- you are taking prescription medications for blood clotting, diabetes, gout, or arthritis. Among those commonly prescribed are Aldactone, Allopurinol, antidepressants, Anturane, Azolid, Butazolidin, Coumadin, Danilone, Diabinese, Dymelor, Hedulin, Heparin, Inderal, Indocin, Indon, Liquamar, Methotrexate, Miradon, Orinase, Oxalid, PABA, Panwarfin, Prednisone, probenecid (Benemid), Sintrom, sulfa drugs, Tandearil, Tofranil, Tolinase, tranquilizers, Tromexan, Zyloprim.
- you have a prior history of allergy, drug sensitivity (particularly to aspirin), or suffer from asthma or asthma-like symptoms.
- you are attempting to relieve the symptoms of arthritis or bursitis.
- you have a history of blood-clotting difficulties.
- you have a history of ulcers.
- you are attempting to treat migraine headaches or headaches from deep within the skull. (Identify them as deep, aching, steady, dull, prolonged.)

- you have recently consumed or will consume alcohol.
- you are attempting to treat aches, pain, or soreness of the body that cannot be related to known injury, strain, or stress.
- on consumption of aspirin or other salicylates, or after a week of self-treatment, symptoms of nausea, vomiting, gastric distress, redness, or itching appear.
- you are attempting to treat symptoms of long duration or ones that exceed the limits described for self-treatment.

If any of these describe your condition, consult your doctor or dentist and your registered pharmacist. Because of their professional training and awareness of your medical history, they can best evaluate and supervise your use of aspirin and its substitutes.

Don't Treat Yourself with Acetaminophen or Phenacetin if—

- you are taking prescription medications for blood clotting such as Coumadin, Danilone, Hedulin, Heparin, Indon, Liquamar, Miradon, Panwarfin, Sintrom, Tromexan.
- the precautions against aspirin and other salicylates (except those referring to allergy, asthma, or ulcers) apply to you.
- you are anemic and plan to take phenacetin.
- you are taking prescribed anticoagulants or oral insulin.

If any of these apply to you, consult your doctor or dentist and pharmacist.

Before Beginning Self-Treatment, It Is Wise to Remember—

- that aspirin and aspirin substitutes relieve certain symptoms but do not cure an ailment.
- to take the manufacturer's advice concerning individual dosage, spacing of doses, and maximum daily dosage unless otherwise directed by your doctor.
- to consult your dentist immediately in case of toothache. Analgesics should only be used for the temporary, emergency relief of such pain.

PRODUCT CHARTS

CHART A: Products Containing *Only* Aspirin or Other Salicylate as Their Pain-Reliever[1]

Key: X—Substance not present; AH—Antihistamine; B—Buffer; S—Mild Stimulant; *—High Salt (Sodium) Content

Brand (Manufacturer)	Delivery Form	Aspirin Content Per Unit	Other Active Ingredients	Intended Rate of Relief[2]	Recommended Single Dose (Adult)[3]
Alka-Seltzer Pain Reliever & Antacid (Miles)	Effer. Tab.	325 mg (5 gr)	Sodium bicarbonate (B);* Citric acid (B)	Rapid	1–2 Tab.
Anacin (Whitehall)	Tab.	400 mg (6.2 gr)	Caffeine (S)	Moderate	1 Tab.
Arthritis Pain Formula (Whitehall)	Tab.	486 mg (7.5 gr)	Aluminum hydroxide (B); Magnesium hydroxide (B)	Moderate	1 Tab.
Arthritis Strength Bufferin (Bristol-Myers)	Tab.	486 mg (7.5 gr)	Aluminum glycinate (B); Magnesium carbonate (B)	Moderate	1 Tab.
A.S.A. (Lilly)	Enseals	325 mg (5 gr)	Enteric coating	Prolonged	1–2 Enseals
		650 mg (10 gr)	Enteric coating	Prolonged	1 Enseal
Ascriptin (Rorer)	Tab.	325 mg (5 gr)	Magnesium hydroxide (B); Aluminum hydroxide (B)	Moderate	1–2 Tab.
Ascriptin A/D (Rorer)	Same as Ascriptin except that buffering content is doubled. Heavy buffering interferes with tetracycline and other antibiotics.				
Aspergum (Plough)	Gum Tab.	228 mg (3.5 gr)	X	Rapid	2 Tab.
Aspirin (Various)	Tab.	325 mg (5 gr)	X	Moderate	1–2 Tab.
Bayer Aspirin (Glenbrook)	Tab.	325 mg (5 gr)	X	Moderate	1–2 Tab.
Bayer Timed-Release Aspirin (Glenbrook)	Capsulated Tab.	650 mg (10 gr)	X	Moderate	1 Tab.

Brand (Manufacturer)	Delivery Form	Aspirin Content Per Unit	Other Active Ingredients	Intended Rate of Relief[2]	Recommended Single Dose (Adult)[3]
Bufferin (Bristol-Myers)	Tab.	325 mg (5 gr)	Aluminum glycinate (B); Magnesium carbonate (B)	Moderate	1–2 Tab.
Congespirin (Bristol-Myers)	Chewable Tab.	81 mg (1.2 gr)	Phenylephrine hydrochloride (Vasoconstrictor)	Rapid	Children: See Label
Fizrin (Glenbrook)	Powder	325 mg (5 gr)	Sodium bicarbonate (B);* Sodium carbonate (B);* Citric acid (B)	Rapid	1–2 Env.
Measurin (Breon)	Time-Rel. Cap.	650 mg (10 gr)	X	Prolonged	1 Tab.
Pabirin (Dorsey)	Tab.	300 mg (4.6 gr)	Aluminum hydroxide (B); Aminobenzoic acid (B)	Moderate	1–2 Tab.
Salicionyl (Upjohn)	Liq.	Sodium salicylate, 650 mg (10 gr)/ 180 ml.	Sodium carbonate (B);* Other buffers	Rapid	90–180 ml.
St. Joseph Aspirin (Plough)	Tab.	325 mg (5 gr)	X	Moderate	1–2 Tab.
St. Joseph Aspirin for Children (Plough)	Chewable Tab.	81 mg (1.2 gr)	X	Rapid	Children: See Label
Uracel (North American)	Tab.	Sodium salicylate, 325 mg (5 gr)*	X	Rapid	1–2 Tab.

1. Use of aspirin or other salicylates is contraindicated in cases of known allergy, anemia, asthma, aspirin hypersensitivity, diabetes, gout, peptic ulcer, and other diseases of the blood or kidney. (See page 9 for possible side effects and drug interactions.)
2. Rapid, moderate and prolonged are relative, descriptive terms.
3. Unless otherwise directed by your doctor. Maximum adult daily dose in self-treatment should not exceed 4.0 g (4,000 mg or 62 gr; see label for children's dosage).

CHART B: Products Containing Combinations of Aspirin, Other Salicylates, Salicylamide, and/or Aminophenols (Acetaminophen/ Phenacetin)[1]

Key: X—Substance not present; AH—Antihistamine; B—Buffer; S—Mild Stimulant; *—High Salt (Sodium) Content; †—"Less than"

Brand (Manufacturer)	Delivery Form	Aspirin or Other Salicylate Content Per Unit	Salicylamide	Acetaminophen
Act-on (Keystone)	Tab.	Sodium salicy-late, 194 mg (3 gr)	130 mg (2 gr)	X
Arthralgen (Robins)	Tab.	X	250 mg (3.9 gr)	250 mg (3.9 gr)
A.S.A. Compound (Lilly)	Tab./ Pluvules	227 mg (3.5 gr)	X	X
Bancap (O'Neal, Jones & Feldman)	Cap.	X	200 mg (3.1 gr)	300 mg (4.6 gr)
Capron (Vitarine)	Cap.	227 mg (3.5 gr)	X	65 mg (1 gr)
Comeback (Norcliff-Thayer)	Tab.	X	150 mg (2.3 gr)	150 mg (2.3 gr)
Dolor (Geriatric Pharmaceutical)	Tab.	230 mg (3.5 gr)	X	230 mg (3.5 gr)
Duradyne (O'Neal, Jones & Feldman)	Tab.	230 mg (3.5 gr)	X	30 mg (.5 gr)
Duragesic (Meyer)	Tab.	Aspirin, 325 mg (5 gr); Salicylsalicylic acid, 163 mg (2.5 gr)	X	X
Empirin Compound (Burroughs Wellcome)	Tab.	227 mg (3.5 gr)	X	X
Excedrin (Bristol-Myers)	Tab.	195 mg (3.0 gr)	130 mg (2 gr)	97 mg (1.5 gr)

Phenacetin	Aspirin Equivalence	Other Active Ingredients	Intended Relief Rate[2]	Recommended Single Dose (Adult)[3]
X	†324 mg †(5 gr)	Sodium bicarbonate (B);* Potassium iodide	Moderate	1–2 Tab.
X	†500 mg †(7.8 gr)	X	Rapid	1 Tab.
160 mg (2.5 gr)	387 mg (6 gr)	Caffeine (S)	Moderate	1–2 Tab.
X	†500 mg †(7.7 gr)	X	Rapid	1 Cap.
162 mg (2.5 gr)	454 mg (7 gr)	Caffeine (S)	Moderate	1 Cap.
X	†300 mg †(4.6 gr)	Caffeine (S)	Rapid	2 Tab.
X	460 mg (7 gr)	Caffeine (S); Calcium carbonate (B)	Moderate	1 Tab.
150 mg (2.3 gr)	410 mg (6.3 gr)	Caffeine (S)	Moderate	1 Tab.
X	488 mg (7.5 gr)	Magnesium hydroxide (B)	Rapid	1 Tab.
162 mg (2.5 gr)	389 mg (6 gr)	Caffeine (S)	Moderate	1 Tab.

Note: Repeated use endangers the kidneys.

X	†422 mg †(6.5 gr)	Caffeine (S)	Rapid	1 Tab.

Chart B: Combination Products

Brand (Manufacturer)	Delivery Form	Aspirin or Other Salicylate Content Per Unit	Salicylamide	Acetaminophen
Excedrin P.M. (Bristol-Myers)	Tab.	195 mg (3 gr)	130 mg (2 gr)	162 mg (2.5 gr)
Goody's Headache Powder (Goody's)	Powder	455 mg (7 gr)	X	X
Maranox (Dent)	Tab.	X	150 mg (2.3 gr)	60 mg (.9 gr)
Medache (Organon)	Tab.	X	150 mg (2.3 gr)	150 mg (2.3 gr)
Nilain (A.V.P.)	Tab.	325 mg (5 gr)	X	163 mg (2.5 gr)
PAC (Upjohn)	Tab.	228 mg (3.5 gr)	X	X
S-A-C (Lannett)	Tab.	X	230 mg (3.5 gr)	150 mg (2.3 gr)
Sal-Fayne (Smith, Miller & Patch)	Cap.	228 mg (3.5 gr)	X	X
S.P.C. (North American)	Tab.	X	195 mg (3 gr)	X
Stanback (Stanback)	a. Tab. b. Powder	a. 325 mg (5 gr) b. 650 mg. (10 gr)/packet	a. 97 mg (1.5 gr) b. 194 mg (3 gr)	X
Trigesic (Squibb)	Tab.	230 mg (3.5 gr)	X	125 mg (1.9 gr)
Vanquish (Glenbrook)	Caplet	227 mg (3.5 gr)	X	194 mg (3 gr)
Zarumin (J.B. Williams)	Tab.	Potassium salicylate, 228 mg (3.5 gr)	260 mg (4 gr)	X

1. Use of combination products can produce the side effects typical of each component.
2. Rapid, moderate, and prolonged are relative, descriptive terms.
3. Unless otherwise directed by your doctor. Maximum daily dose in self-treatment should *not* exceed manufacturer's warning.

Phenacetin	Aspirin Equivalence	Other Active Ingredients	Intended Relief Rate[2]	Recommended Single Dose (Adult)[3]
X	†487 mg †(7.5 gr)	Methylpyri- lene fumarate (AH)	Rapid	1 Tab.
33 mg (.5 gr)	488 mg (7.5 gr)	Caffeine (S)	Rapid	1 Env.
100 mg (1.5 gr)	†310 mg †(4.7 gr)	Caffeine (S)	Rapid	2 Tab.
X	300 mg (4.6 gr)	Caffeine (S); Phenyltolox- amine (AH)	Rapid	2 Tab.
X	488 mg (7.5 gr)	Caffeine (S)	Moderate	1 Tab.
163 mg (2.5 gr)	391 mg (6 gr)	Caffeine (S)	Moderate	1 Tab.
X	†380 mg †(5.8 gr)	Caffeine (S)	Rapid	1–2 Tab.
166 mg (2.6 gr)	394 mg (6.1 gr)	Caffeine (S)	Moderate	1 Tab.
130 mg (2 gr)	†325 mg †(5 gr)	Caffeine (S)	Rapid	1–2 Tab.
X	a.†422 mg †(6.5 gr) b.†844 mg †(13 gr)	Caffeine (S)	Rapid	a. 1 Tab. b. 1 Packet exceeds Rec. Max. Dose
X	355 mg (5.4 gr)	Caffeine (S)	Moderate	1 Tab.
X	421 mg (6.5 gr)	Aluminum hydroxide (B); Magnesium hydroxide (B); Caffeine (S)	Moderate	1 Caplet
X	†488 mg †(7.5 gr)	X	Rapid	1 Tab.

Chart C: Products Containing Only Aminophenols (Acetaminophen)[1]

Key: X—Substance not present; AH—Antihistamine; B—Buffers; S—Mild Stimulant; *—High Salt (Sodium) Content

Brand (Manufacturer)	Delivery Form	Acetaminophen Content Per Dose	Other Active Ingredients	Intended Rate of Relief[2]	Recommended Single Dose (Adult)[3]
Acetaminophen Uniserts (Upsher-Smith)	Suppos.	a. 125 mg (1.9 gr) b. 300 mg (4.6 gr) c. 600 mg (9.2 gr)	X	Moderate	a. Children: See Label b. 1 Suppository c. 1 Suppository
Amphenol (O'Neal, Jones & Feldman)	Tab.	325 mg (5 gr)	X	Moderate	1–2 Tab.
Apamide (Dome)	Tab.	300 mg (4.6 gr)	X	Moderate	1–2 Tab.
Bayer Non-Aspirin Pain Reliever (Glenbrook)	Tab.	325 mg (5 gr)	X	Moderate	1–2 Tab.
Bromo-Seltzer (Warner-Lambert)	Effer. Granules	325 mg (5 gr)	Phenacetin, 130 mg (2 gr)/ capful; Caffeine (S); Sodium bicarbonate (B);* Citric acid (B)	Rapid	1 Capful
Datril Analgesic (Bristol-Myers)	Tab.	325 mg (5 gr)	X	Moderate	1–2 Tab.
Dularin Syrup (Dooner)	Liq.	240 mg/10 ml (3.7 gr)	X	Rapid	20 ml (Children: See Label)
Febrinol (Vitarine)	Tab.	325 mg (5 gr)	X	Moderate	1–2 Tab.
Liquiprin (Norcliff-Thayer)	Liq.	240 mg/5 ml (3.7 gr)	X	Rapid	Children: See Label
Nebs (Eaton)	a. Tab. b. Liq.	a. 325 mg (5 gr) b. 240 mg/ 10 ml (3.7 mg)	a. X b. Alcohol, 7%	a. Moderate b. Rapid	a. 1–2 tab. b. 15–20 ml (Children: See Label)
Percogesic (Endo)	Tab.	325 mg (5 gr)	Phenyltoloxamine (AH)	Moderate	1–2 Tab.

Brand (Manufacturer)	Delivery Form	Acetaminophen Content Per Dose	Other Active Ingredients	Intended Rate of Relief[2]	Recommended Single Dose (Adult)[3]
SK-APAP (Smith Kline & French)	a. Tab.	a. 325 mg (5 gr)	a. X	a. Moderate	a. 1–2 Tab.
	b. Liq. (Elixir)	b. 240 mg/10 ml (3.7 gr)	b. Alcohol, less than 10%	b. Rapid	b. 15–20 ml (Children: See Label)
St. Joseph Fever Reducer for Children (Plough)	a. Drops	a. 80 mg/ .8 ml (1.2 gr)	a. Alcohol, less than 10%	a. Rapid	a. See Label
	b. Liq.	b. 120 mg/ 5 ml (1.8 gr)	b. Alcohol, less than 8%	b. Rapid	b. See Label
Tempra (Mead-Johnson)	a. Tab.	a. 325 mg (5 gr)	a. X	a. Moderate	a. 1–2 Tab. (Adults)
	b. Syrup	b. 130 mg (2 gr)/tsp	b. Alcohol, 10%	b. Rapid	b. Children: See Label
	c. Drops	c. 65 mg (1 gr)/ ½ tsp	c. Alcohol, 10%	c. Rapid	c. Children: See Label
Tenol (North American)	Tab.	325 mg (5 gr)	X	Moderate	1–2 Tab.
Tylenol (McNeil)	a. Tab.	a. 325 mg (5 gr)	a. X	a. Moderate	a. 1–2 Tab.
	b. Drops	b. 60 mg (1 gr)/ dropper	b. Alcohol, less than 8%	b. Rapid	b. Children: See Label
	c. Liq.	c. 120 mg (1.9 gr)/ 5 ml (tsp)	c. Alcohol, less than 8%	c. Rapid	c. Children: See Label
	d. Chewable Tab.	d. 120 mg (1.9 gr)	d. X	d. Rapid	d. Children: See Label
Tylenol Extra Strength (McNeil)	Tab.	500 mg (7.7 gr)	X	Moderate	1 Tab.
Valadol (Squibb)	a. Tab.	a. 325 mg (5 gr)	a. X	a. Moderate	a. 1–2 Tab.
	b. Liq. (Elixir)	b. 120 mg (1.8 gr)/ 5 ml (tsp)	b. Alcohol, 9%	b. Rapid	b. Children: See Label

1. Aminophenols are generally recommended substitutes for aspirin, other salicylates, and combination products in cases of known allergy, asthma, anemia, aspirin hypersensitivity, diabetes, gout, peptic ulcer, and other digestive disorders. (See page 11 for side effects and drug interactions.)
2. Rapid, moderate, and prolonged are relative, descriptive terms.
3. Unless otherwise directed by your doctor. Maximum adult daily dose in self-treatment should *not* exceed 2.6 g (2,600 mg. or 40 gr; see label for children's dosage).

2
COLDS
COUGHS
ALLERGIES
ASTHMA
SINUSITIS

GENERAL CONSIDERATIONS

It is easy to confuse the common cold with coughs, allergies, sinusitis, or asthma. Although their symptoms are similar, their origins are quite different. Effective treatment requires awareness of those differences. An antihistamine is apt to relieve the nasal stuffiness of an allergy. It will probably have little effect on the nasal stuffiness of a cold.

The Common Cold

Cause and Effect Of the more than 125 different viruses that can cause a cold, more than 60 primarily attack the lining of your nose. They produce the nasal discharge, stuffiness, and congestion of a "head cold." Others may concentrate on the lining of the throat, the bronchial passages, or the larynx. Before the typical cold has run its course (7–14 days), all the membranes of your nose, throat, and bronchial passages may be affected.

First symptoms generally involve the "target" organ. A runny nose (*rhinorrhea*), sneezing, and/or throat discomfort are typical signs of onset. These symptoms tend to disappear as your nasal discharge or mucus becomes thick and heavy. The resulting sense of stuffiness may extend into your sinuses to cause headaches and into your lungs to cause chest congestion and coughing. Lethargy, muscular ache, and feverishness (although there is usually little or no actual fever) are typical of a fully developed cold.

Because initial symptoms closely resemble those of more serious diseases, you must observe them carefully. A fever, severe sore throat, and/or a rash are *not* typical. In the presence of other cold symptoms, they may mean the start of pneumonia, measles, flu, tonsillitis, strep throat, chicken pox, or German measles. Contact your doctor if an actual fever lasts more than 24–36 hours, if your throat is genuinely sore rather than dry or irritated, if a skin rash appears, or if any symptoms are particularly severe.

Treatment Because the common cold is rarely serious and is usually limited in duration, self-treatment is reasonable. The most immediate and sensible measures include bed rest (particularly during the first 24–48 hours), proper nutrition (to maintain the body's defenses), generous fluid intake (to dilute congestion), and increasing the humidity of the air you breathe (to soothe irritated membranes of your nose, throat, and vocal cords). Medication is a supplement to this basic therapy but can only relieve, *not* cure, your symptoms.

Nasal discharge, stuffiness, and congestion A runny nose is common at the start of a cold. Stuffiness and congestion usually follow. Using a surface and/or an oral decongestant can ensure a proper flow of air and help you avoid irritation from excessive nose-blowing. *Topical (surface) decongestants* (sprays, drops, jellies, or inhalants) act rapidly to reduce swelling and drip. They provide only temporary relief. If used too often (beyond recommended dosages) or for too long (more than 3–4 days), they can cause "rebound congestion" with intense swelling of the nasal membranes and thickening of the mucus. *Oral decongestants* act more slowly, with less impact, but for longer periods than topical forms. Because they are carried by your bloodstream, they may cause side effects that are not triggered by surface decongestants. If you have high blood pressure, hypertension, hyperthyroidism, or take MAO inhibitors (a type of antidepressant), you should avoid oral decongestants unless otherwise advised by your doctor.

Antihistamines have little or no effect on the nasal stuffiness of a cold, and taking them when they are not needed doesn't make sense. Unfortunately, many cold remedies contain a combination of nasal decongestants and antihistamines. Careful use of a topical and an oral decongestant in recommended dosages will probably give you the safest and most effective relief from a runny nose or nasal stuffiness.[1]

Sore throat (pharyngitis) A dry and irritated sore throat may respond to the soothing action of sugar, a hard candy, proper humidification (increasing water vapor in the air you breathe with a vaporizer or a pot of boiling water), or a salt gargle. By soothing the throat, you may relieve irritation and suppress your impulse to cough. Antibacterial[2] mouthwashes, gargles, or cough drops are not effective in treating cold symptoms, which are produced by a virus. Surface anesthetics[3] in some cough drops may reduce the cough impulse, but be careful since the

---

1. The anticholinergics (atropine and belladonna alkaloids) can produce a drying of the nasal passageways; however, their side effects are probably too serious to warrant inclusion in self-treatment.
2. Cetylpyridinium chloride is the usual antibacterial agent.
3. Benzocaine is the usual anesthetic agent.

anesthetic effect may mask symptoms of more serious disease. The inclusion of a cough suppressant along with an anesthetic in some lozenges is generally recognized as safe, but the amount of suppressant is usually not enough to be effective. Since "soreness" in a child is hard to measure, getting your pediatrician's advice is wise.

Hoarseness (laryngitis)   Your vocal cords are located at the top of your windpipe and cannot be reached by gargles, washes, or cough drops. Treat hoarseness by resting your voice, proper humidification, and avoiding smoke, dust, and volatile fumes.

Coughs without congestion   A dry, hacking, or irritable cough that is repetitive and produces little phlegm usually occurs at the beginning of a cold. Throat irritation often triggers it. Soothing your throat (see above) and/or mildly depressing your nervous system may relieve the impulse to cough. *Oral suppressants (antitussives)* inhibit the cough reflex. Both narcotic (codeine) and non-narcotics (dextromethorphan and diphenhydramine) have been judged safe and effective for this purpose. At recommended dosages there is little chance of codeine addiction, although a tendency to constipation may occur. Products containing these ingredients should be avoided if you suffer from a chronic pulmonary disease (asthma or emphysema) or shortness of breath, or by children taking other drugs. Diphenhydramine is a powerful antihistamine, which may cause either drowsiness or excitability (particularly in children). It should not be taken if you have glaucoma or prostate difficulty and in general by children under 6.

Coughs with chest congestion (bronchitis)   A congested cough, which may or may not produce heavy mucus (phlegm or sputum), is typical of a developed cold. It serves the important function of expelling fluid from the lungs. If your cough produces mucus or phlegm, it is probably useful and should not be suppressed. The fluids carried into the throat and mouth will generally soothe the lining of the passageways and prevent your cough from becoming hyperactive. Increasing the humidity of the air you breathe is helpful. If your cough is congested but does not produce mucus or phlegm, it is not relieving your lungs of fluid. Using an oral cough suppressant for a congested but non-productive cough doesn't make sense. Failure to eject the congestion is usually a result of its being too thick, and drinking plenty of liquids (water, juice, etc.) can thin it. In theory *expectorant* drugs, which are present in most cough remedies, also thin congestion, but the FDA's Advisory Review Panel has found no expectorant to be both safe and effective for this purpose.

The inclusion of a single oral decongestant with a single cough suppressant is reasonable in combination cold products, but including antihistamines (other than diphenhydramine) in cough remedies is of dubious merit.

Headache, fever, and malaise   Headaches associated with a cold usually come from sinus pressure and can frequently be relieved by deconges-

tants. Any fever lasting more than 24–36 hours or one of more than 100°
F. requires your doctor's advice and supervision. The use of aspirin or an
aspirin substitute may give you immediate relief from headache,
feverishness, or muscular ache. Because you should not be using aspirin
if you have a history of asthma, allergy, high blood pressure, kidney
disease, peptic ulcer, or diabetes (see Chapter 1), acetaminophen in dosages of 325 mg (5 gr) to 650 mg (10 gr) is often the drug to choose. Both
aspirin and acetaminophen are frequently included in combination products which can reasonably be taken if your concurrent symptoms include headache, low-grade fever, and/or muscular ache.

Secondary Infections   Although the common cold tends to be self-
limiting, it can lead to other infections, e.g., pneumonia and ear infections, or sinusitis (see below). If a cold lasts more than 10 days, or if you
have a high fever, severe symptoms, or hearing loss, consult your doctor
immediately.

Coughs

A cough is one of your body's natural defense mechanisms. It rids the
lungs, windpipe, and throat of foreign objects, particles, or fluids. The
cough reflex generally begins with irritation of the sensitive membranes along the lower respiratory tract. In the common cold, the impulse usually starts with mucus in your lungs or a dry, irritated throat.
In typical allergies, stimulus comes from dust, pollen, animal dandruff,
or a postnasal drip which overflows into your throat or lungs. Coughs,
which may be indistinguishable from those of a cold or allergy, can be
voluntary or result from smoking, asthma, emphysema, or heart disease. Because of their many possible origins, treat your cough symptoms
with care. Consult your doctor if any cough lasts more than 10 days or if
you also have a fever, difficulty breathing, or bloody sputum. Don't use a
cough suppressant when you have chest congestion.

Allergies

Cause and Effect   Airborne pollens from ragweed, grasses, and/or
trees; dust; smoke; animal dandruff; flour; grains; seeds; detergents;
and/or other agents may inflame the tissues lining your nose and throat.
As many as 30 million Americans are sensitive to the irritation caused
by one or more of these agents (allergens).[1] Inflammation begins on

---

1. Although susceptibility is not strictly inherited, a predisposition runs in families, with
onset most frequent in children, less so in adolescents, and least in adults.

contact. Because most allergens are airborne, it is the lining of your nose that is most vulnerable. Susceptible cells respond to the allergen by releasing a substance called *histamine* that causes nasal blood vessels to swell and to produce a watery mucus. Swelling (*edema*), runny nose (*rhinorrhea*), and stuffiness are all typical of a nasal allergy (*allergic rhinitis*). Other typical symptoms are paroxysms of sneezing, itching (*pruritus*) of the nose and eyes, and tearing. If your contact with the allergen continues, mucus may overflow into the chest or throat (post-nasal drip) causing irritation and congestion that eventually produce a cough. Your eyes may redden and headache may develop as congestion spreads into the sinuses and creates pressure. The symptoms remain as long as the susceptible nasal tissue is in contact with the allergen.

The concentration of grass and tree pollen is highest during the spring, while ragweed pollen is at its peak concentration in the later summer and early fall. If you are sensitive to pollen, you suffer from *seasonal rhinitis,* a disorder which you can usually identify by its recurrence at the same time each year and treat with non-prescription drugs. Other allergens tend to be present continuously throughout the year and cause a more serious allergy, *perennial rhinitis,* whose persistent irritation may seriously injure the nasal tissue. This condition needs your doctor's attention. A major difference between seasonal and perennial allergies is that seasonal rhinitis usually begins with sneezing, followed by a runny nose and stuffiness, whereas attacks of perennial rhinitis tend to begin with congestion and postnasal drip. If the normally watery mucus becomes thick, a secondary bacterial infection is probably occurring and you should get to your doctor immediately.

Treatment Complete avoidance of the offending allergen is ideal but rarely possible. Using face masks and air conditioner filters and avoiding vegetation and open windows can lessen the severity of seasonal allergies.

Antihistamines When taken orally these drugs block the effects of histamine and can reduce swelling and control a runny nose for up to 8 hours. They also limit sneezing, itching, and tearing. Postnasal drip is slowed and the likelihood of a cough is reduced.

Because the antihistamines generally depress your nervous system, drowsiness is a common side effect, and you must avoid situations requiring alertness (driving a car or operating machinery). Although the sedative effect varies among the antihistamines, take none if you are using alcohol or are under a doctor's care using prescription drugs. Your doctor's advice is also necessary if you take antihistamines and have asthma, glaucoma, or urinary retention, or if you are treating a child under 6. Although such sensitivity is rare, children with a tendency to convulsive disorders may become excited, irritable, or suffer insomnia when taking antihistamines.

Oral antihistamines at recommended dosages are the primary ingredients of choice for self-treatment. The topical antihistamines found in some sprays, drops, and lozenges are of questionable effectiveness because they generally do not penetrate inflamed tissue.

Decongestants   Nasal sprays, drops, inhalants, and jellies rapidly reduce the swelling of inflamed membranes and the flow of mucus. Although relief from your symptoms is dramatic, it is only temporary and invites excessive medication. Overuse (either at higher dosages, with greater frequency, or for longer periods than recommended) may lead to severe "rebound congestion," which may be more intense than the original stuffiness.

The action of _oral decongestants_ is slower and less intense, but may relieve symptoms without causing "rebound congestion." Because they cause constriction of blood vessels throughout the body, your use of oral forms requires your doctor's supervision in treating children under 6 or if you have high blood pressure, hypertension, a heart condition, or hyperthyroidism. Although the combination of an antihistamine and an oral decongestant is not advisable for treating the common cold, such a combination is reasonable for treating nasal allergies.[1]

Cough suppressants and expectorants   To have a cough along with symptoms of an allergy is relatively rare, but may result if postnasal drip irritates the lining of your throat. Although antihistamines should control the drip, the use of a cough suppressant without an expectorant may help you control the dry, hyperactive cough that may develop. If your cough is congested, it may indicate a more serious allergic condition or secondary infection, in which case you should see your doctor.

Analgesics   Although allergies rarely cause headaches, aspirin or acetaminophen in 325–650 mg (5–10 gr) dosages may relieve the symptom if it appears. Because acetaminophen produces fewer side effects and negative drug interactions, it is usually the drug to choose (see Chapter 1). Although aspirin or an aspirin substitute has the approval of the FDA's Advisory Review Panel as a combination ingredient, you are wiser to take a single-ingredient analgesic separately from other medication and only when needed.

Lozenges, gargles, and mouthwashes   The soothing action of sugar may relieve throat irritation and inhibit your impulse to cough. The inclusion of a local anesthetic will more certainly relieve irritation but may mask the symptoms of a severe sore throat. It is more reasonable to use antiseptics and antibacterials in the treatment of an allergy than in colds since secondary bacterial infection is more likely with allergies. However, the concentrations of these ingredients in non-prescription products are generally too low to be effective.

---

1. The anticholinergics (atropine and belladonna alkaloids) can produce a drying of the nasal passageways, but their side effects are probably too serious to warrant inclusion in self-treatment.

Secondary Infection Prolonged or severe allergic reactions may lead to more serious disease. Congestion forced into the ears can cause inflammation (*otitis*) and bacterial infection. Congestion forced into the sinuses may produce a chronic inflammation (*sinusitis*) along with headache and the growth of polyps. As many as 30% of those who suffer from allergic rhinitis later develop bronchial asthma. Initial symptoms, which include a tightening in the chest and a slight wheezing, require immediate consultation with your doctor.

Asthma

At least 5 million Americans suffer from asthma. Aspirin, an allergic reaction, a respiratory infection, or emotional stress may trigger a seizure. Symptoms of attack, which may last from a few minutes to a few hours, typically begin with chest constriction, followed by increasingly severe cough, shortness of breath, and an acute sense of suffocation. Mucus tends to be thick.

Treatment Non-prescription medications containing bronchodilators (ephedrine, epinephrine, methoxyphenamine, and theophylline) cause tightened air passages to expand, thereby relieving acute distress. Although these compounds are generally recognized as safe and effective, the seriousness of asthma requires that your doctor supervise their use. Don't diagnose or treat asthma on your own.

Sinusitis

Intense or prolonged nasal congestion can impair the drainage of your sinuses. Inflammation often results and can cause headache, tenderness, and/or facial pain. Careful self-treatment with topical and/or oral decongestants may ease the blockage, while careful use of analgesics should relieve headache or pain. Call your doctor if the mucus becomes thick, if fever appears, or if pain is intense.

SELF-TREATMENT

The common cold and seasonal allergies produce many similar symptoms. Intelligent self-treatment begins by knowing which one is causing your discomfort.

You Probably Have a Cold if—

- your symptoms include some combination of a runny nose (rhinorrhea), nasal congestion, mild to moderate throat discomfort, sneezing, cough (hacking or deep), hoarseness, chest congestion, headache, and/or general lethargy, aches, and pains.
- the onset of your symptoms has been gradual (1–2 days) with sneezing, scratchy throat, and/or runny nose occurring before heavy congestion, headache, or cough.
- your cold symptoms occur in the late fall or midwinter. Although spring and summer colds are not uncommon, spring and late summer are the peak periods for seasonal allergies.
- your cold symptoms are not too severe, particularly in terms of throat discomfort and fever, and if no rash or intense breathing difficulty is noted.
- you do not have a history of allergy, asthma, bronchitis, emphysema, or heart disease.

You Probably Have an Allergy if—

- your symptoms include a combination of sneezing, itching of nose and eyes, tearing, runny nose, and/or postnasal drip.
- you or your family (parents, brothers, or sisters) has a history of allergy or asthma.
- your symptoms are more or less continuous throughout the year (perennial allergic rhinitis) or reappear seasonally in the spring or late summer (seasonal allergic rhinitis).
- the onset of your symptoms has been rapid or spontaneous, beginning either with sneezing and a runny nose (seasonal) or nasal congestion and postnasal drip (perennial).
- your symptoms have tended to reappear over the years or tend to recur when you stop medication.

You Probably Have Another Condition if—

- you have a fever of 100° F. or more.
- any fever lasts more than 24–36 hours.
- you have a severe sore throat.
- the watery mucus of a suspected allergy becomes thick, if hearing becomes impaired, if a congested cough develops, or if you feel chest constriction.
- the mucus contains blood.

- a skin rash appears at any time.
- you have symptoms other than those described, if a cold lasts more than 7–14 days, or if an allergy persists beyond 10 days.

If any of these apply to you, consult your doctor.

Self-Treatment of the Common Cold

- Self-treatment is reasonable so long as you are not run down, pregnant, or suffering from unusually severe symptoms, other disease conditions, or secondary complications—in which case, see your doctor.
- Bed rest, well-balanced meals, plenty of fluids, and ample humidification of the air you breathe are the basis for intelligent care.
- Medications can do nothing but relieve some of the unpleasant symptoms of your cold until it has run its natural course.

Self-Treatment of Allergic Rhinitis

- If your allergy can be related to such environmental changes as weather, climate, or geography (seasonal allergy), self-treatment is generally appropriate so long as you are not run down, pregnant, nor suffering from another chronic or acute disease.
- If your allergy persists throughout the year (perennial allergy), self-treatment is not wise. Such chronic irritation requires your doctor's supervision.
- Avoidance of the irritant allergen is the ideal.
- Non-prescription medications can do nothing but relieve some of the unpleasant symptoms of your allergy.

General Guidelines for Self-Treatment of the Common Cold and Seasonal Allergies

- Treat only the symptoms you have and not ones you anticipate.
- Treat a symptom only as long as it lasts.
- Treat each symptom individually. Try to use a product that contains a single, appropriate, safe and effective active ingredient.
- Consult your registered pharmacist to be sure that the active ingredient(s) in any product is present in the right amount *per dose* to relieve your specific symptom(s).
- Use a product containing a minimum of different active ingredients. If you use a fixed-combination product, be sure that each

active ingredient is safe, effective, and appropriate to one of your symptoms.
- Don't use a product for children unless the label has specific instructions about children's dosages.
- Avoid products that combine 2 active ingredients intended for the treatment of a single symptom, e.g., 2 or more antihistamines, 2 or more decongestants, etc.
- Avoid products that combine more than 3 kinds of active ingredients.
- Avoid products that contain active ingredients which are apt to produce side effects or adverse reactions in you.
- Avoid products that do not indicate the amounts of each active ingredient on the label.

The Symptoms of a Common Cold and Active Ingredients for Their Relief

SYMPTOM	YOU CAN USE
Runny nose and stuffiness (swelling and congestion)	Decongestant sprays, drops, inhalants, or jellies; oral decongestants; or oral anticholinergics (see note 5)
Coughs	
a. frequent, dry, and hacking	a. Cough suppressants (antitussives)
b. infrequent, congested and producing mucus	b. Proper humidification and ample fluid intake
c. infrequent, congested and not producing mucus	c. Oral expectorants with or without a cough suppressant (see notes 3, 4)
Headache, malaise, and/or low-grade fever	Aspirin, acetaminophen, or other aspirin substitute
Dry or irritated throat; also, indirectly, for coughs	Topical anesthetics or antibacterials (see note 6); expectorants (see note 4); hard candy; or salt-water gargle
Hoarseness	Proper humidification and resting of the vocal cords
Chest congestion	Oral decongestants; bronchodilators; or expectorants (see note 4)

NOTES

1. Antihistamines are not suitable for the relief of cold symptoms.
2. Topical and oral decongestants used carefully in combination are generally effective.
3. Cough suppressants are only appropriate for frequent and hacking coughs not complicated by congestion.
4. In theory expectorants could be useful in diluting your chest congestion. In practice the FDA Advisory Review Panel has yet to find any expectorant with proven effectiveness.
5. Anticholinergics are not recommended for relieving symptoms of congestion because of the serious side effects they may produce.
6. Topical anesthetics, as in cough drops, may mask the symptoms of a severe sore throat. Topical antibacterials, also in cough drops, are of little or no use in treating a viral disease such as a cold.
7. Fixed-combination cold products can be recommended for self-treatment if the product contains only one kind of active ingredient for each symptom, if the amount of each active ingredient is present in effective dosages, if each active ingredient is generally regarded as safe and effective, and if each active ingredient is appropriate for a different and concurrent symptom.

The Symptoms of a Seasonal Allergy and Active Ingredients for Their Relief

SYMPTOM	YOU CAN USE
Any combination of runny nose or stuffiness, sneezing, itch, tearing, etc.	An oral antihistamine
Runny nose and stuffiness	Decongestant sprays, drops, inhalants, and jellies; oral decongestants; or oral anticholinergics (see note 5)
Headache	Aspirin, acetaminophen, or other aspirin substitute
Irritated throat	Topical anesthetics, antibacterials or expectorants (see note 5)
Chest congestion	Oral decongestants or oral bronchodilators

NOTES

1. The principal medication for relief of all symptoms is a single ingredient antihistamine (oral).

2. Topical decongestants can provide rapid and effective short-term relief from a runny nose and nasal stuffiness, but be careful not to use them at more than recommended dosages or for more than 3–4 days.
3. Oral decongestants are effective over longer periods than topical decongestants. Using a single ingredient topical decongestant *and* a single ingredient oral decongestant is reasonable.
4. Aspirin, acetaminophen, or other aspirin substitute may be used individually or in combination with other ingredients if you have a headache.
5. No anticholinergic nor expectorant has been found both safe and effective at recommended dosages.
6. Fixed-combination allergy products are recommended for self-treatment if the product contains only one kind of active ingredient for each symptom, if the amount of each active ingredient is present in effective dosages, if each active ingredient is right for one of your different and concurrent symptoms, and if each active ingredient is generally regarded as safe and effective.

Classes of Medically Active Ingredients Used in Cold Remedy and Allergy Products[1]

Cough Suppressants (Antitussives)

Indicated use   For temporary suppression of the impulse to cough.
Contraindications   In the presence of heavy chest congestion typical of a severe cold, asthma, bronchitis, or emphysema; in the presence of a high fever, rash, or persistent headache; if a cough lasts more than 7 days; in children under 2. (Consult your doctor.)

Look for Ingredients Generally Judged Safe and Effective:
Oral Codeine, Dextromethorphan, and Diphenhydramine.
   Codeine may produce nausea or constipation. It is not for use if you have a chronic pulmonary disease or shortness of breath, or by children taking other drugs. Dextromethorphan may cause drowsiness or upset stomach. Diphenhydramine may make you sleepy or excitable. It is not for use by children under 6, or if you have glaucoma or urinary difficulty. Consult your registered pharmacist about recommended dosage.

Active ingredients generally judged safe but of uncertain effectiveness   Creosote, ethylmorphine hydrochloride (reacts like codeine; see box above for possible problems), and noscapine hydrochloride.
   Other claimed cough suppressants judged safe but of uncertain effectiveness include camphor (topical/inhalant), caramiphen edisylate, car-

---

1. Based on the FDA Advisory Review Panel Report, published in the *Federal Register*, September 9, 1976.

betapentane citrate, cod-liver oil, elm bark, eucalyptol (topical/inhalant), thymol (topical/inhalant), and turpentine.

Avoid all other ingredients.

Expectorants
Indicated use   To temporarily reduce the thickness of phlegm so it may be cleared from the lungs and respiratory passageways. Soothing action may help reduce the impulse to cough.

Ingredients Generally Judged Safe and Effective: None.

Active ingredients generally judged safe but of uncertain effectiveness
Ammonium chloride (may cause nausea, vomiting, or severe indigestion and is not to be used if you have a heart, kidney, or lung disease), glyceryl guaiacolate (Guaifenesin), ipecac syrup, potassium guaiacolsulfonate, and terpin hydrate.

Other claimed expectorants judged safe but of uncertain effectiveness include creosote, benzoin compounds, camphor (inhalant), eucalyptol, menthol, pine tar products, sodium citrate, tolu products, and turpentine oil.

Ingredients generally judged unsafe and/or ineffective include antimony potassium tartrate; chloroform; iodides of calcium, lime, or potassium; ipecac fluidextract; squill; and turpentine oil (oral).

Antihistamines
Indicated use   For the temporary relief of symptoms associated with a seasonal allergy (runny nose, stuffiness, sneezing, itching of eyes and nose, tearing, and postnasal drip).

Contraindications   In the treatment of a common cold; if you have bronchial asthma, glaucoma, or urinary retention; in situations where you must be alert (driving and the operation of machinery); by children under 12; in conjunction with alcohol, anticoagulants, hypnotics, sedatives, or antianxiety drugs. (Consult your doctor.)

Possible side effects and adverse reactions   With the exception of phenindamine, which is a stimulant, the antihistamines are nervous system depressants that may produce drowsiness. Excessive doses may have the opposite effect: restlessness, insomnia, and/or excitability. Dryness of the mouth is frequent. Blurred vision and mild constipation are possible.

Look for Ingredients Generally Judged Safe and Effective:
Brompheniramine, Chlorpheniramine, and Pheniramine (least sedative).
Methapyrilene, Pyrilamine, and Thonzylamine (moderately sedative).
Diphenhydramine and Doxylamine (most sedative).
Phenindamine (may cause restlessness or excitation).
Consult your registered pharmacist about recommended dosages.

Ingredients generally judged safe but of uncertain effectiveness Phenyltoloxamine and thenyldiamine.

Nasal Decongestants

Indicated use For the temporary relief of nasal discharge, stuffiness, and congestion associated with *either* the common cold or allergy.

Topical forms (nasal sprays, drops, inhalants, jellies) For rapid and pronounced, though temporary, relief of symptoms.

Oral forms (solid or liquid) For more prolonged though less intense relief of symptoms, particularly when "rebound congestion" (intensified congestion caused by reaction to the drug) is a possibility.

Contraindications to topical forms If used for more than 3–4 days, excessive application may lead to absorption into the bloodstream from the stomach or produce "rebound congestion."

Contraindications to oral forms For children under 6; if you have high blood pressure, heart disease, diabetes, or hyperthyroidism; if you are taking such prescription drugs as Butonyl, Furoxone, Marplan, Matulane, Nardil, Niamid, Niconyl, Nydrazid, or Parnate. (Consult your doctor.)

Look for Ingredients Generally Judged Safe and Effective:
Topical Ephedrine compounds, Naphazoline, Oxymetazoline, Phenylephrine, and Xylometazoline; Oral Phenylephrine, Phenylpropanolamines, and Pseudoephedrines; and Inhalant Propylhexedrine.
Consult your registered pharmacist about recommended dosages.

Ingredients generally judged safe but of uncertain effectiveness Oral ephedrine and topical phenylpropanolamine.

Other claimed decongestants generally judged as safe but of uncertain effectiveness include bornylacetate (topical), camphor (topical/inhalant), cedarleaf oil (topical), creosote, 1-desoxyephedrine (inhalant), eucalyptol (topical/inhalant), menthol (topical/inhalant), thenyldiamine (topical), thymol (inhalant), and turpentine oil (topical/inhalant).

Ingredients generally judged unsafe or ineffective Mustard oil and oral turpentine.

Anticholinergics (Atropine and Belladonna Alkaloids)

Indicated use Relief of excessive nasal discharge and eye secretions typical of hay fever, allergic rhinitis, and the common cold.
Contraindications The FDA Advisory Review Panel does not find either atropine or belladonna alkaloids effective for treatment at dosages considered safe. Their use is not recommended.

Aspirin and Aspirin Substitutes The pain-reducing (analgesic) effect of aspirin or acetaminophen can relieve the headache and malaise associated with the common cold or allergy. The FDA Advisory Review Panel approves the use of combination products containing aspirin or aspirin substitute if headache or malaise is a concurrent symptom. (See Chapter 1 for a full consideration of these drugs.)

Other Ingredients Included in Cold Remedies and Products for the Treatment of Seasonal Allergy

Vitamin C The effectiveness of vitamin C (ascorbic acid) in preventing or relieving the symptoms of a common cold has not been established. According to proponents of vitamin C therapy, 1–5 grams per day is necessary for prevention and up to 15 grams per day is necessary for relief once symptoms appear. No non-prescription cold remedy currently contains dosages exceeding 200 mg and most contain 20–50 mg. These dosages are too small to be effective and consumption of vitamin C in fixed-combination remedies is probably unreasonable. If you choose to use ascorbic acid in large quantity, select a product that contains only that vitamin. In large doses you may experience diarrhea. The concurrent use of aspirin or an anticoagulant drug may be harmful.
Caffeine Non-prescription products frequently contain caffeine to counteract the drowsiness that antihistamines may cause. The amount present in most combinations is less than that in a quarter cup of coffee. The FDA Advisory Review Panel, while judging these amounts of caffeine safe, finds little or no evidence for its effectiveness or rationale for its inclusion.
Alcohol Many cough syrups and liquid antihistamine/decongestant products contain alcohol to help dissolve other ingredients. Concentrations range from 1% to 42%. Children, diabetics, and those taking sedative, hypnotic, antidepressant, and/or antianxiety medications should avoid products with more than minimal percentages of alcohol.

PRODUCT CHARTS

CHART A: A Selected List of Cold and Allergy Medications

Brand (Manufacturer)	Delivery Form	Antihistamine[1]	Decongestant	Analgesic[2]	Other Active Ingredients[3]
Alka-Seltzer Plus (Miles)	Tab.	Chlorpheniramine, 1 mg	Phenylephrine, 7.8 mg	X	Sodium bicarbonate, 1.6 g (AA)
Allerest (Pharmacraft)	a. Tab. b. Chewable Tab. for Children	a. Chlorpheniramine, 1 mg; Methapyrilene, 5 mg b. Chlorpheniramine, .5 mg; Methapyrilene, 2.5 mg	a. Phenylpropanolamine, 25 mg b. Phenylpropanolamine, 12.5 mg	X	X
Allerest (Pharmacraft)	Time-Rel. Cap.	Methapyrilene, 10 mg; Pyrilamine, 15 mg	Phenylpropanolamine, 50 mg	X	X
BC All Clear (Block)	Powder	Chlorpheniramine, 2 mg	Phenylephrine, 10 mg	Aspirin, 645 mg; Salicylamide, 195 mg	Caffeine, 32.4 mg
Chlor-Trimeton (Schering)	a. Tab. b. Syrup	a. Chlorpheniramine, 4 mg b. Chlorpheniramine, 2 mg/tsp.	X	X	a. b. Alcohol, 7% X
Cold-Team-24 (Chesebrough-Pond)	Tab.	X	Phenylpropanolamine, 25 mg	Aspirin, 650 mg	Caffeine, 30 mg
Contac (Menley & James)	Time-Rel. Cap.	Chlorpheniramine, 4 mg	Phenylpropanolamine, 50 mg	X	Belladonna, .2 mg (AC)

Colds, Coughs, Allergies, Asthma, and Sinusitis   39

CHART A: A Selected List of Cold and Allergy Medications

Brand (Manufacturer)	Delivery Form	Antihistamine[1]	Decongestant	Analgesic[2]	Other Active Ingredients[3]
Coricidin "D" (Schering)	Tab.	Chlorpheniramine, 2 mg	Phenylephrine, 10 mg	Aspirin, 389 mg	Caffeine, 32.4 mg
Coricidin Demilets (Schering)	Chewable Tab. for Children	Chlorpheniramine, .5 mg	Phenylephrine, 2.5 mg	Aspirin, 80 mg	X
Coricidin Medilets (Schering)	Chewable Tab. for Children	Chlorpheniramine, .5 mg	X	Aspirin, 80 mg	X
Coryban-D (Roerig)	Cap.	Chlorpheniramine, 2 mg	Phenylpropanolamine, 25 mg	Salicylamide, 365 mg	Caffeine, 30 mg; Vit. C, 25 mg
Co-Tylenol Cold Formula (McNeil)	Tab.	Chlorpheniramine, 1 mg	Phenylephrine, 5 mg	Acetaminophen, 325 mg	X
Dristan (Whitehall)	Cap.	Chlorpheniramine, 4 mg	Phenylephrine, 20 mg	X	X
Dristan (Whitehall)	Tab.	Phenindamine, 9.6 mg	Phenylephrine, 5 mg	Aspirin, 325 mg	Caffeine, 15.5 mg; Aluminum & Magnesium antacids
Listerine (Warner-Lambert)	Tab.	X	Phenylpropanolamine, 25 mg	Acetaminophen, 325 mg	Caffeine, 32.5 mg
Neo-Synephrine Compound (Winthrop)	Tab.	Thenyldiamine, 7.5 mg	Phenylephrine, 5 mg	Acetaminophen, 150 mg	Caffeine, 15 mg

Product	Form	Antihistamine	Decongestant	Analgesic	Other
Neo-Synephrine, Elixir (Winthrop)	Liq.	X	Phenylephrine, 5 mg/tsp	X	Alcohol, 8%
Novahistine Fortis (Dow)	Cap.	Chlorpheniramine, 2 mg	Phenylephrine, 10 mg	X	X
Ornex (Smith Kline & French)	Cap.	X	Phenylpropanolamine, 18 mg	Acetaminophen, 325 mg	X
Sinarest (Pharmacraft)	Tab.	Chlorpheniramine, 1 mg	Phenylephrine, 5 mg	Acetaminophen, 300 mg	Caffeine, 30 mg
Sine-Aid (Johnson & Johnson)	Tab.	X	Phenylpropanolamine, 25 mg	Aspirin, 324 mg	X
Sucrets Cold Decongestant (Calgon)	Lozenge	X	Phenylephrine, 5 mg; Phenylpropanolamine, 10 mg	X	Benzocaine, 5 mg (Anesthetic)
Sudafed (Burroughs Wellcome)	Tab. Liq.	X	Pseudoephedrine, 30 mg/tab or tsp	X	X
Super Anahist (Warner-Lambert)	Tab.	Phenyltoloxamine, 6.25 mg; Thonzylamine, 6.25 mg	Phenylpropanolamine, 12.5 mg	Aspirin, 227 mg; Phenacetin, 97 mg	Caffeine, 32.4 mg
Triaminic (Dorsey)	Time-Rel. Cap.	Pheniramine, 25 mg; Pyrilamine, 25 mg	Phenylpropanolamine, 50 mg	X	

1. Whether the antihistamine is in the form of a hydrochloride, maleate, fumarate, etc., is not of great significance.
2. See Chapter 1 for a full discussion of aspirin and aspirin substitutes.
3. Antacid (AA); Anticholinergic (AC)

Brand (Manufacturer)	Del. Form	Antitussive (Cough Suppressant)	Decongestant	Expectorant[1]	Antihistamine/ Other[2]
Arrestin Extra Strength (Mitchum-Thayer)	Liq.	Dextromethorphan, 10 mg/tsp	X	G. guaiacolate, 25 mg	Alcohol, 10%; Sodium citrate, 50 mg (E)
Benylin (Parke-Davis)	Liq.	X	X	X	Diphenhydramine, 12.5 mg/tsp (AH)
Breacol (Glenbrook)	Liq.	Dextromethorphan, 10 mg/tsp	Phenylpropanolamine, 38 mg/tsp	X	Chlorpheniramine, 4 mg/tsp (AH); Alcohol, 10%
Cerose (Ives)	Cap.	Dextromethorphan, 10 mg	Phenylephrine, 7.5 mg	Terpin hydrate, 65 mg	Chlorpheniramine, 2 mg (AH); Acetaminophen, 194 mg (A); Vit. C, 25 mg
Cheracol (Upjohn)	Liq.	Codeine, 11 mg/tsp	X	G. guaiacolate, 115 mg/tsp	X
Cheracol D (Upjohn)	Liq.	Dextromethorphan, 60 mg/2 tbl	X	G. guaiacolate, 77.5 mg/2 tbl	X
Cidicol (Upjohn)	Liq.	Ethylmorphine, 15.5 mg/2 tbl	X	Guaiacolsulfonate, 500 mg/2 tbl	X
Cold-Team-Nighttime (Chesebrough-Pond)	Liq.	Dextromethorphan, 30 mg/2 tbl	Phenylephrine, 10 mg/2 tbl	X	Chlorpheniramine, 2 mg/2 tbl (AH); Acetaminophen, 600 mg/2 tbl (A)

Product	Form	Antitussive	Decongestant	Expectorant	Other
Coryban-D (Roerig)	Liq.	Dextromethorphan, 7.5 mg/tsp	Phenylephrine, 5 mg/tsp	G. guaiacolate, 50 mg/tsp	Acetaminophen, 120 mg/tsp (A); Vit. C, 12.5 mg/tsp
Creomulsion (Creomulsion)	Liq.	X	X	Creosote, .03 ml/tbl; Ipecac, .04 ml/tbl	Cascara, Menthol, White pine, Wild cherry
Deka Expectorant (Winthrop)	Liq.	Codeine, 9.2 mg/tsp	X	Squill, 11 mg/tsp; Tolu balsam, 86 mg/tsp	X
Dondril Anticough (Whitehall)	Tab.	Dextromethorphan, 10 mg	Phenylephrine, 5 mg	G. guaiacolate, 50 mg	Chlorpheniramine, 1 mg (AH)
Dristan (Whitehall)	Liq.	Dextromethorphan, 150 mg/tsp	Phenylephrine, 100 mg/tsp	G. guaiacolate, 600 mg/tsp	Chlorpheniramine, 20 mg/tsp (AH)
Elixir Terpin Hydrate (Upjohn)	Liq.	Codeine, 60 mg/2 tbl	X	Terpin hydrate, 480 mg/2 tbl	Alcohol, 40%
Listerine Big 4 (Warner-Lambert)	Liq.	Dextromethorphan, 15 mg/2 tbl	Phenylpropanolamine, 37.5 mg/2 tbl	G. guaiacolate, 100 mg/2 tbl	Chlorpheniramine, 2 mg/2 tbl (AH)
Norwich Elixir (Norwich)	Liq.	Dextromethorphan, 65 mg/2 tbl	X	Terpin hydrate, 500 mg/2 tbl	Alcohol, 42%
Novahistine DH (Dow)	Liq.	Codeine, 10 mg/tsp	Phenylephrine, 10 mg/tsp	X	Chlorpheniramine, 2 mg/tsp (AH)
Novahistine Expectorant (Dow)	Liq.	Codeine, 10 mg/tsp	Phenylephrine, 10 mg/tsp	G. guaiacolate, 100 mg/tsp	Chlorpheniramine, 2 mg/tsp (AH)

CHART B: A Selected List of Cough Remedies (Antitussives)

Brand (Manufacturer)	Del. Form	Antitussive (Cough Suppressant)	Decongestant	Expectorant[1]	Antihistamine/Other[2]
Nyquil (Vick)	Liq.	Dextromethorphan	Ephedrine	X	Doxylamine (AH); Acetaminophen, 600 mg (A); Alcohol, 25%
Orthoxicol (Upjohn)	Liq.	Dextromethorphan, 10 mg/tsp	Methoxyphenamine, 17 mg/tsp	X	X
Pertussin 8-Hr. (Chesebrough-Pond)	Liq.	Dextromethorphan, 30 mg/20 ml	X	X	Alcohol, 9.5%
Robitussin (Robins)	Liq.	X	X	G. guaiacolate, 100 mg/tsp	X
Robitussin-PE (Robins)	Liq.	X	Phenylephrine, 10 mg/tsp	G. guaiacolate, 100 mg/tsp	X
Romilar III (Sauter)	Liq.	Dextromethorphan, 5 mg/tsp	Phenylpropanolamine, 12.5 mg/tsp	G. guaiacolate, 50 mg/tsp	Alcohol, 10%
Romilar for Children (Sauter)	Chew. Tab.	Dextromethorphan, 7.5 mg	X	X	Benzocaine, 20 mg (Anesthetic)
St. Joseph for Children (Plough)	Liq.	Dextromethorphan, 7.5 mg/tsp	X	X	Menthol, .5 mg/tsp; Sodium citrate, 100 mg/tsp (E)
Triaminic Expectorant (Dorsey)	Liq.	X	Phenylpropanolamine, 12.5 mg/tsp	G. guaiacolate, 100 mg/tsp	Pheniramine, 6.25 mg/tsp (AH); Pyrilamine, 6.25 mg/tsp (AH)
Vicks Formula 44 (Vick)	Liq.	Dextromethorphan	X	X	Doxylamine (AH); Sodium Citrate; Alcohol, 10%

1. Glyceryl: G
2. Analgesic (A); Claimed expectorant (E); Antihistamine (AH)

CHART C: A Selected List of Topical (Nasal) Decongestants

Brand (Manufacturer)	Del. Form	Decongestant	Antiseptic	Antihistamine & Other Active Ingredients[1]
Afrin (Schering)	Drops Spray	Oxymetazoline, .05%	Benzalkonium chloride, .02%	X
Allerest (Pharmacraft)	Spray	Phenylephrine, .5%	Benzalkonium chloride, .02%	Methapyrilene, .2% (AH)
Benzedrex (Smith Kline & French)	Inhaler	Propylhexedrine, 250 mg	X	Menthol, 12.5 mg, & other aromatic oils
Coryban-D (Roerig)	Spray	Phenylephrine, .5%	X	X
Dristan (Whitehall)	Mist Spray	Phenylephrine, .5%	Benzalkonium chloride	Pheniramine, .2% (AH); Aromatic oils
Mentholatum (Mentholatum)	Oint.	X	Boric Acid, 9%	Menthol, Camphor, & other aromatic oils
Neo-Synephrine (Winthrop)	a. Drops b. Jelly c. Spray	Phenylephrine: a. 1%, .5%, .25%, .125% b. .5% c. .5%, .25%	Benzalkonium chloride	Various aromatic oils
NTZ (Winthrop) *Also* NTR	Drops Spray	Phenylephrine, .5%	Benzalkonium chloride	Thenyldiamine, .1% (AH)
Otrivin (Ciba-Geigy)	Drops Spray	Xylometazoline, .1%	X	X
Otrivin Pediatric (Ciba-Geigy)	Drops Spray	Xylometazoline, .05%	X	X
Privine (Ciba-Geigy)	Drops Spray	Naphazoline, .05%	Benzalkonium chloride	X
Spec-T Sore Throat (Squibb)	Spray	X	X	Benzociane, 2% (Anesthetic)
Triaminicin (Dorsey)	Spray	Phenylpropanol-amine, .75%; Phenylephrine, .25%	Benzalkonium chloride	Pheniramine, .125% (AH); Pyrilamine, .125% (AH)
Vicks Sinex (Vick)	Spray	Phenylephrine	Cetylpyridinium	Methapyrilene (AH); Aromatic oils

1. Antihistamine (AH)

Colds, Coughs, Allergies, Asthma, and Sinusitis   45

3
INSOMNIA
TENSION
FATIGUE

GENERAL CONSIDERATIONS

Sleep and Sleeplessness

Insomnia may involve problems of falling asleep or of remaining asleep. Difficulty in relaxing interferes with your getting to sleep. Any tension, overstimulation, restlessness, anxiety, physical pain, or discomfort can keep you awake. Changes in biological rhythms, which occur with age, may cause you to wake up once you have fallen asleep. Chronic pain or illness, depression, or the use of drugs that interfere with specific phases of the sleep cycle (especially dreaming) can have the same effect. Awaking early is characteristic of the elderly or the anxiety-ridden.

Self-Treatment of Insomnia

Trouble in falling or remaining asleep is usually a temporary problem and self-treatment is generally appropriate. If the difficulty is severe enough to impair daytime activities seriously or so chronic that it occurs for at least 10 consecutive nights, consult your doctor. Such insomnia may indicate serious underlying illness.

Medication (Nighttime Sleep-Aids) Certain antihistamines are the only potentially safe and effective non-prescription drugs for encouraging sleep. Single ingredient products containing methapyrilene, pyrilamine, or phenyltoloxamine are currently available. Single ingredient products containing diphenhydramine or doxylamine may be marketed in the near future. Fixed-combination products containing more than 2 antihistamines or antihistamine(s) in combination with ammonium, potassium or sodium bromides; scopolamine, scopolamine aminoxide, or scopolamine hydrobromide; citric acid, passionflower extract, sodium bicarbonate, thiamin, niacinamide, vitamin C (ascorbic acid), or other ingredients should *not* be used for self-treatment. It is reasonable to use aspirin or an aspirin substitute in combination with an antihistamine *only* if simple pain, e.g., headache or toothache, is keeping you awake.

Using Daytime Sedatives for Tension, Stress, and Anxiety

A host of different factors, ranging from comparatively simple psychological or physical pressures to severe emotional or organic disease may cause tension, stress, or anxiety. Because the range of possible causes is so great, the wisdom of treating yourself with non-prescription products is questionable. Acute attacks of anxiety, depression, or hysteria require immediate medical attention. Chronic nervousness, stress, or tension also need a doctor's supervision. Treating yourself over a period of time may mask serious disease and produce severe side effects or psychological addiction, while putting off needed professional treatment. The accurate self-diagnosis of mild and transient tension is difficult.

Self-Treatment of Tension, Stress, and Anxiety

Non-prescription products that claim to provide relief from "simple" nervous tension have not met FDA standards for effectiveness. The antihistamines that have provisional approval as nighttime sleep-aids offer serious drawbacks for daytime use—the drowsiness they often produce is welcome in helping put you to sleep but may be dangerous during waking hours when alertness is desirable. Other active ingredients commonly included in daytime sedatives are unsafe or ineffective (bromides or scopolamine compounds) or are inappropriate (ascorbic acid, citric acid, niacinamide, sodium bicarbonate, aspirin or aspirin substitute).

Drowsiness, Fatigue and Alcoholic Hangover

Overwork is probably the least frequent cause of fatigue, while anxiety, depression, frustration, and boredom are probably the most common. More rarely, glandular imbalance, anemia, infection, circulatory disease, or low blood sugar may be responsible for symptoms of tiredness or exhaustion.

Enthusiasm and interest are the most effective factors in overcoming drowsiness or fatigue, but such natural stimulants cannot always be supplied at will, particularly if a task is both prolonged and tedious, e.g., driving long distances or preparing income tax forms. The use of limited quantities of caffeine (up to 200 mg/3–4 hours) in such instances can safely and effectively stimulate greater alertness and mental acuity. In such quantities caffeine heightens central nervous system function and improves the tone of skeletal muscles.

Most of us take caffeine by drinking a cup of coffee (100–150 mg), a cup of tea (50–75 mg), or a cola drink (40–60 mg/8 oz.). Dosages larger than 250 mg often produce insomnia, restlessness, irritability, headache, and/or heartbeat irregularities. These symptoms may be mistaken for temporary anxiety neurosis in amounts exceeding 1 gram (1000 mg) per day (8–10 cups of coffee).

Taking caffeine as an antidote to alcohol is not advisable. Although caffeine may counteract the drowsiness associated with recent drinking, judgment remains impaired and you are no less inebriated. After a few hours the effects of alcohol in the bloodstream may become stimulative. Caffeine can add to the effect and may lead to stomach upset.

Self-Treatment with Non-Prescription Stimulants Single ingredient (caffeine) non-prescription products are suitable for promoting alertness while you are doing tedious work. Use them only occasionally, in recommended dosages, and not along with coffee, tea, or cola drinks. The recommended dosage is 100–200 mg every 3–4 hours. Avoid combination products containing ingredients other than caffeine (ammonium chloride, ginseng, vitamin E, etc.).

SELF-TREATMENT

Self-Treatment with a Nighttime Sleep-Aid May Be Appropriate in Recommended Dosages if—

- you have *occasional* trouble falling asleep.
- you have *occasional* trouble remaining asleep.

Self-Treatment with a Nighttime Sleep-Aid Is Probably Not Advisable if—

- your insomnia is severe (example: impairs normal daytime activities).
- your insomnia is chronic (example: persists every night for 10 days to 2 weeks).

- acute pain, shortness of breath, cough, asthma, indigestion, frequent urination, or any other symptom of a chronic disease keeps you from falling asleep or remaining asleep.
- you are pregnant or nursing a baby.
- you suffer from glaucoma, heart disease, peptic ulcer, or prostate difficulty.
- you simultaneously use alcohol or prescription drugs that depress the central nervous system.

Before You Choose to Treat Insomnia Yourself, Consider the Possible Causes of Your Sleeplessness

- Have you consumed more caffeine than usual (coffee, tea, or cola drinks)?
- Have you been taking prescription drugs that may produce overstimulation as a side effect (Ritalin, Tenuate, Preludin, Dexedrine, or other amphetamine)?
- Have you been using drugs that may interfere with normal sleep patterns e.g., alcohol, barbiturates, tranquilizers, antidepressants, or reserpine? Withdrawal may produce wakefulness or "rebound dreaming" (usually nightmares) that can interfere with your rest.
- Have you been taking naps?
- Have you had a recent shift in your normal sleeping and waking schedule?
- Have you been experiencing unusual stress or tension? If so, will it be temporary or prolonged?
- Has your sleep been interrupted by headache, pain, difficulty in breathing, or need to urinate? (Consult your doctor.)
- Have you tried such other inducements to sleep as a warm bath, milk, hot toddy, eye shades, ear plugs, or deep breathing?
- Have you been getting adequate exercise?

If You Decide to Use a Nighttime Sleep-Aid, Be Aware—

- that such medication is intended for the relief of occasional sleeplessness in adults. Do not give such medication to a child under 12.
- that such drugs are not advisable if you are pregnant or nursing a baby.
- that you should discuss the simultaneous use of prescription drugs and sleep-aids with your doctor or registered pharmacist.

- that if your symptoms last more than 10 days to 2 weeks, a serious underlying disease may be the cause and you should consult your doctor.
- that the only potentially safe and effective ingredient is an antihistamine.
- that the simultaneous use of alcohol isn't sensible.

How to Select or Evaluate a Nighttime Sleep-Aid

The FDA Advisory Review Panel on Nighttime Sleep-Aids, Daytime Sedatives, and Stimulants[1] concludes that many of the ingredients commonly included in sleep products are neither safe nor effective for use in the self-treatment of occasional sleeplessness. Others are judged unreasonable. Only specific antihistamines in recommended doses are considered *potentially* safe and effective. Although the safety and effectiveness of these antihistamines is not seriously in question, they must undergo at least three years of further testing before they can receive full approval. During this time they will probably remain available for non-prescription use.

Because of the stringency of the FDA Panel's recommendations, many products may change their composition by eliminating dangerous components. Judge a product from its label in terms of the following:

- Choose only single ingredient products containing *only one* of the following antihistamines: Methapyrilene (fumarate or hydrochloride), Pyrilamine maleate, Diphenhydramine,[2] Doxylamine,[2] Phenyltoloxamine. The possible side effects of these antihistamines include dizziness, dryness of the mouth and throat, blurred vision, stomach upset, and irritability (particularly in children). Cease medication and consult your doctor if any of these symptoms appear.
- Avoid any product that does not identify its medically active ingredients and their concentrations.
- Avoid any product containing ammonium, potassium, or sodium bromides.
- Avoid any product containing scopolamine, scopolamine hydrobromide, or scopolamine aminoxide.
- Avoid any product containing citric acid, passionflower extract, niacinamide, vitamin C (ascorbic acid), or any ingredient other

---

1. *Federal Register,* December 8, 1975
2. Not marketed as a sleep-aid at this writing

than one of the antihistamines listed above and, possibly, aspirin or an aspirin substitute.

- Avoid all combination products except a combination containing a safe and effective antihistamine compounded with aspirin or an aspirin substitute (acetaminophen, phenacetin, or salicylamide) in recommended dosage strength. Use a product containing both an antihistamine and an analgesic *only* if mild to moderate pain is the source of your insomnia.

Self-Treatment with a Daytime Sedative Is Medically Questionable

- "Tension," unlike insomnia, cannot be easily defined.
- The symptoms of tension have many different origins and degrees of severity. Therefore, no simple, safe, and effective dosage of a mood-altering drug can be recommended.
- Substituting a daytime sedative for alcohol is dangerous.
- The only potentially safe and effective daytime sedative products *may* be ones containing a single ingredient antihistamine. However, the sleep-promoting side effect, which makes an antihistamine useful for insomnia, may produce drowsiness during daytime activities. Driving a car or operating machinery while taking such medication is risky.
- The FDA Advisory Review Panel sees no benefits from such medication and has recommended that all daytime sedative products bear the following warning: "This product has not been demonstrated to be effective to the satisfaction of the FDA."

Self-Treatment with a Stimulant—

- may be reasonable on an occasional basis.
- may be safe and effective when used to reduce the fatigue or tedium associated with long, boring, and repetitive tasks.

Self-Treatment with Non-Prescription Stimulants Is Not Advisable—

- in treatment of alcoholic hangover or as an antidote to alcohol consumption.
- in conjunction with coffee, tea, or cola drinks.
- in dosages exceeding 100–200 mg of caffeine every 3–4 hours. Disturbances such as anxiety, irritability, insomnia, or heartbeat irregularities may occur at higher dosages.
- for children under 12.
- for self-treatment lasting more than 7–10 days.

How to Select or Evaluate a Stimulant Product

- Choose only single ingredient products containing caffeine.
- Avoid all combination products. (Typical secondary ingredients to be avoided include ginseng, ammonium chloride, and vitamin E.)

PRODUCT CHARTS

CHART A: A Selected List of Sleep-Aids and Sedatives

Brand (Manufacturer)	Delivery Form	Antihistamine[1]	Other Active Ingredients[2]
Compoz (Jeffrey Martin)	Tab.	Methapyrilene, 15 mg; Pyrilamine, 10 mg	Scopolamine aminoxide, .15 mg (AC)
Dilone (Endo)	Tab.	Phenyltoloxamine, 30 mg	Acetaminophen, 325 mg (A); Caffeine, 30 mg (S)
Excedrin P.M. (Bristol-Myers)	Tab.	Methapyrilene, 25 mg	Aspirin, 194.4 mg (A); Acetaminophen, 162 mg (A); Salicylamide, 129.6 mg (A)
Nervine (Miles)	Cap. Liq. Tab.	Methapyrilene, 25 mg	X
Nytol (Block)	a. Cap. b. Tab.	a. Methapyrilene, 50 mg b. Methapyrilene, 25 mg	a. Salicylamide, 380 mg (A) b. Salicylamide, 200 mg (A)
Percogesic (Endo)	Tab.	Phenyltoloxamine, 30 mg	Acetaminophen, 325 mg (A)
Placin Calmative (Commerce)	Cap.	X	Salicylamide, 186 mg (A); Aminobenzoic acid, 62 mg
Quiet World (Whitehall)	Tab.	Methapyrilene, 17 mg	Scopolamine hydrobromide, .083 mg (AC); Aspirin, 219 mg (A); Acetaminophen, 156 mg (A)
Sleep-Eze (Whitehall)	Tab.	Methapyrilene, 25 mg	Scopolamine hydrobromide, .125 mg (AC)
Sominex (J. B. Williams)	a. Cap. b. Tab.	a. Methapyrilene, 50 mg b. Methapyrilene, 25 mg	a. Scopolamine hydrobromide, .50 mg (AC); Salicylamide, 200 mg (A) b. Scopolamine hydrobromide, .25 mg (AC); Salicylamide, 200 mg (A)

1. Antihistamines are marketed in the form of citrates, fumarates, hydrochlorides, or maleates. These formulations should have little effect on your evaluation or selection.
2. Pain-reliever (A), see Chapter 1; Stimulant (S); Anticholinergic (AC)

CHART B: A Selected List of Stimulant Products

Brand (Manufacturer)	Del. Form	Caffeine	Other Active Ingredients[1]
Double-E (Keystone)	Cap.	180 mg	Thiamin hydrochloride, 5 mg (V)
No-Doz (Bristol-Myers)	Tab.	100 mg	X
Pre-Mens Forte (Blair)	Tab.	100 mg	Ammonium chloride, 500 mg (D)
Prolamine (Thompson)	Cap.	140 mg	Phenylpropanolamine hydrochloride, 35 mg (AH)
Tirend (Norcliff-Thayer)	Tab.	100 mg	X
Vivarin (J. B. Williams)	Tab.	200 mg	Dextrose, 150 mg (S)

1. Antihistamine (AH); Diuretic (D); A sugar (S); Vitamin (V)

4
THE DIGESTIVE SYSTEM

Acid Indigestion

GENERAL CONSIDERATIONS

Eating rapidly, indiscreetly, or under tension often produces symptoms of excess stomach acid (hyperacidity or acid indigestion). A burning sensation in your throat or chest may indicate that stomach acid has flowed upward into your esophagus or food pipe. The corrosive action of this digestive fluid irritates the sensitive esophageal lining and causes heartburn. Overproduction of normal stomach acids may result from tension, anxiety, or overeating. These excess acid concentrations can penetrate the mucous lining that ordinarily protects the stomach wall. Symptoms of burning, aching, gnawing, pressure, or pain in your abdomen commonly indicate a sour stomach. Self-treatment for occasional episodes of such distress is probably reasonable as long as your discomfort is not complicated by other symptoms, chronic disease, certain medications, and/or a medical history that suggests possible complications.

Complicating Factors

Over extended periods of time excess stomach acid may produce peptic ulcers. In such cases, symptoms of recurrent heartburn, sour stomach, and/or acid indigestion are typical and tend to occur regularly, e.g., before or after meals. Because any ulcerative condition is dangerous, even life-threatening, your self-treatment of such known, suspected, or potential distress[1] is unwise. Indeed, prolonged treatment of any excess acid symptom is hazardous and should not continue for longer than 2 weeks without your doctor's advice and supervision. Get medical help at once if vomiting occurs or if stools are black and tarry. Your doctor's guidance is also needed if acidity is severe, particularly if it is accompanied by

---

1. Although peptic ulcers are not inherited, the tendency to develop them is.

shortness of breath, sweating, and/or actual chest pain. Acid indigestion in combination with these symptoms may indicate an impending heart attack. Other severe diseases which may be signaled by acid indigestion include gastritis, hiatus hernia, cancer of the stomach or small intestine, and diseases of the pancreas.

Principles of Self-Treatment

To block or neutralize the chemical activity of stomach acid is the goal of self-treatment. Although any substance that counteracts acid activity may be called an antacid, bases or alkalizing agents neutralize acids most directly and are the principal antacids available for self-treatment. Aluminum (carbonate, phosphate, or hydroxide), calcium (carbonate or phosphate), magnesium (carbonate, hydroxide, oxide, or trisilicate), and sodium (carbonate or bicarbonate) are among the most common alkalizing agents found in non-prescription products. Other substances (attapulgite, carboxymethylcellulose, kaolin, methylcellulose, or pectin) may effectively reduce acidic irritation by absorbing digestive acids. Alginic acid may prevent digestive acids from flowing upwards into the esophagus and producing heartburn, while simethicone may lessen the pain or discomfort of gas (flatulence), which can accompany acid indigestion. None of these active ingredients has been shown to coat or soothe stomach linings, nor to affect symptoms of nervous or emotional disturbances, excessive smoking, food intolerance, colds, nervous tension headaches, or the morning sickness of pregnancy. They can only neutralize or counteract the stomach acidity of indigestion, heartburn, or a sour stomach.

All antacid agents are capable of producing side effects after prolonged or excessive use. The risks are minimal if self-treatment is temporary and you don't exceed recommended dosages.

Simultaneous use of any prescription drug and an antacid may cause neither to have its desired effect. An antacid greatly reduces the effectiveness of many antibiotics, particularly tetracycline, penicillin, and the sulfonamides. Similar interference can occur with anticoagulants, pentobarbital, cortisone, and other antiarthritic medications. Before selecting an antacid, consult your doctor or registered pharmacist about possible drug interactions.

Delivery Forms
Liquids and suspensions   These give the most rapid and certain relief since the active ingredients offer the greatest surface area and medium for chemical interaction.
Tablets and gums   You must thoroughly chew and dissolve these forms to achieve maximum surface area for chemical interaction. Since com-

plete disintegration or dissolving is uncertain, acid neutralizing effects may be reduced.

Effervescent powders Because the gas produced by effervescence may compound your discomfort, completely dissolve these forms in water until all gas production ceases.

SELF-TREATMENT

Self-Treatment with an Antacid May Be Advisable if—

- your symptoms involve only *temporary* acid indigestion following excessive eating.
- your symptoms of overindulgence are heartburn or sour stomach.
- the symptoms you wish to treat occur very seldom.
- your symptoms include a headache. You may reasonably use an antacid in combination with a pain reliever (aspirin or aspirin substitute).
- your symptoms are accompanied by gas. You may reasonably use an antacid in combination with an antiflatulent (simethicone).

Self-Treatment with an Antacid Is Probably Not Advisable if—

- any single episode of "indigestion" is severe, particularly if you experience shortness of breath, sweating, and/or chest pain.
- vomiting occurs.
- stools are black and tarry.
- your symptoms are recurrent (more than once or twice a month) or are regular (before or after meals).
- you or your family (parents, brothers, or sisters) has a history of peptic ulcers.
- you suffer from heart or kidney disease (gout, stones, urinary retention, etc.), hypertension, or swelling (particularly of the legs and ankles).
- you are taking any prescription medication (particularly tetracycline, penicillin, sulfonamides, pentobarbital, anticoagulants,[1] isoniazid, cortisone or other antiarthritic medication). Consult your doctor or registered pharmacist for advice.
- you suffer from constipation or diarrhea *before* beginning medication.
- your symptoms become more severe after self-treatment or persist for more than 2 weeks.

Treating yourself with an antacid on a regular basis can be risky. Symptoms of a serious disease may be masked or serious side effects

---

1. Except warfarin

may develop. Consult your doctor if symptoms continue or increase or if any listed contraindications apply to you.

How to Select or Evaluate an Antacid Product

In June of 1974 the FDA published a monograph which rigorously defines the appropriate uses of antacids in self-treatment, classifies medically active ingredients according to safety and effectiveness, indicates appropriate dosages, and lists requirements for proper labeling. Products that do not conform to stated criteria must be altered or withdrawn from the marketplace. A number of compounds having one or more ingredients now judged as safe but of uncertain effectiveness must have their efficacy proved within a fixed period of time.

Because many antacid medications did not originally meet all standards for safety, effectiveness, and proper dosage strength, reformulation of many familiar products is occurring rapidly. Be certain to check product labels for changes in content, formulation, and/or dosage. Follow all recommendations concerning appropriate use, dosage strength, possible side effects and drug interactions. Remember that all recommendations apply *only to the occasional use* of these products. Many antacid ingredients that are safe and effective for temporary self-treatment become hazardous with prolonged or excessive use.

Antacid Ingredients Considered both Safe and Effective

The principal antacid ingredient in any product you select should be one or more of the following:

- Aluminum (carbonate, phosphate, or hydroxide)
- Bismuth (aluminate, carbonate, subcarbonate, subgallate, or subnitrate)
- Calcium (carbonate or phosphate)
- Citric Acid
- Dihydroxyaluminum (aminoacetate, aminoacetic acid, or sodium carbonate)
- Glycine (aminoacetic acid)
- Hydrated magnesium aluminate
- Magaldrate
- Magnesium (carbonate, glycinate, hydroxide, oxide, or trisilicate; see note 2)
- Milk solids (dried)
- Sodium (bicarbonate, carbonate, or potassium tartrate; see notes 2, 3)
- Tartaric acid (tartrate salt)

1. In most product categories combinations of 2 or more medically active ingredients with the same function, e.g., 2 antihistamines, are considered unreasonable. However, with antacids the combination of 2 or more acid-neutralizing ingredients, e.g., aluminum and magnesium hydroxides, can be reasonable and even desirable.
2. Magnesium and potassium can be poisonous if you have a kidney disorder. Read the label—it will warn you of potentially dangerous concentrations of these elements—and avoid them unless your doctor tells you otherwise.
3. The sodium content of some antacid products can be harmful if you are on a salt-free or salt-restricted diet. The label will warn you if you should avoid such products.
4. Some antacid ingredients (aluminum and calcium compounds) may be constipating while others (magnesium compounds) may produce diarrhea. The tendency to cause either of these side effects is noted on product labels. Such compounds may contain other ingredients to counteract these problems.

Antacid Ingredients Considered Safe but of Uncertain Effectiveness

Products may contain these ingredients until their effectiveness has been determined: alginic acid, attapulgite, carboxymethylcellulose, kaolin, methylcellulose, pectin, and simethicone.

NOTES It is claimed that—

1. alginic acid may prevent stomach acid from flowing into the esophagus and producing heartburn.
2. attapulgite, carboxymethylcellulose, kaolin, methylcellulose, and pectin may absorb excess acid and prevent it from harming the stomach lining.
3. simethicone may lessen the pain or pressure of gas (flatulence).

Combinations of Active Ingredients

1. Products may reasonably contain 2 or more active, safe, and effective antacid components.
2. Products may reasonably contain antacid(s) and aspirin or an aspirin substitute for the simultaneous relief of acid indigestion and headache. Use such a compound only if you have *both* symptoms.
3. Use a product containing antacid(s) and an antiflatulent (simethicone) only if symptoms of acid indigestion and gas (flatulence) occur together.

PRODUCT CHART

A Selected List of Antacids

Brand (Manufacturer)	Delivery Form	Aluminum Hydroxide	Calcium Carbonate	Magnesium Oxide, Hydroxide, or Trisilicate	Other Active Ingredients[2]
Alka-2 (Miles)	Chew. Tab.	X	500 mg	X	X
Alka-Seltzer Effervescent Antacid (Miles)	Effer. Tab.	X	X	X	Citric acid, 800 mg; Potassium bicarbonate, 300 mg; Sodium bicarbonate, 1000 mg
Alkets (Upjohn)	Tab.	X	750 mg	65 mg	Magnesium carbonate, 130 mg
Aludrox (Wyeth)	a. Tab. b. Liq.	a. 233 mg b. 297 mg/tsp	X	a. 83.5 mg b. 96 mg	(S) (S)
Amphojel (Wyeth)	a. Tab. b. Liq.	a. 300 mg b. 250 mg/tsp	X	X	(S) (S)
A-M-T (Wyeth)	a. Tab. b. Liq.	a. 150/mg b. 246 mg/tsp	X	a. 250 mg[1] b. 625 mg/tsp[1]	(S) (S)
Basaljel (Wyeth)	a. Tab. b. Cap. c. Liq.	a. 500 mg b. 500 mg c. 400 mg/tsp	X	X	(S) (S) (S)
Bell-Ans (Dent)	Tab.	X	X	X	Sodium bicarbonate, 264 mg; Charcoal; Ginger

Brand (Manufacturer)	Delivery Form	Aluminum Hydroxide	Calcium Carbonate	Magnesium Oxide, Hydroxide, or Trisilicate	Other Active Ingredients[2]
Bisodol (Whitehall)	Tab. Powder	X	188 mg	172 mg Hydroxide; 55 mg Trisilicate	(S)
Camalox (Rorer)	Tab. Liq.	225 mg/tab or tsp	250 mg/tab or tsp	200 mg/tab or tsp	X
Chooz (Plough)	Gum Tab.	X	356 mg	162 mg[1]	X
Creamalin (Winthrop)	Tab.	320 mg	X	75 mg	(S)
Delcid (Merrell-National)	Liq.	600 mg/tsp	X	665 mg/tsp	X
Dicarbosil (Lewis-Howe)	Tab.	X	489 mg	X	(S)
Di-Gel (Plough)	a. Tab. b. Liq.	a. 282 mg b. 245 mg/tsp	X	85 mg/tab or tsp	Simethicone, 25 mg/tab or tsp; (S)
Eno (Beecham)	Powder	X	X	X	Sodium bicarbonate (7.6%), Citrate (27.2%), Tartrate (65.2%)
Fizrin (Glenbrook)	Powder	X	X	X	See chart A, Chap. 1
Gelusil (Warner-Chilcott)	a. Tab. b. Liq.	a. 250 mg b. 267 mg/4 ml	X	a. 500 mg[1] b. 515 mg/4 ml[1]	a. (S) b. Alginic acid, 48 mg/4 ml; (S)
Gelusil Flavor Pak (Warner-Chilcott)	Liq.	267 mg/4 ml	X	515 mg/4ml[1]	X

Gelusil-Lac (Warner-Chilcott)	Powder	1000 mg	X	2000 mg[1]	Milk solids; (S)
Gelusil-M (Warner-Chilcott)	a. Tab. b. Liq.	a. 250 mg b. 265 mg/tsp	X	a. 100 mg Hydroxide; 500 mg Trisilicate b. 104 mg Hydroxide; 515 mg Trisilicate/tsp	a. (S) b. Alginic acid, 60 mg/tsp; (S)
Haley's M-O (Sterling)	Liq.	X	X	75%	Mineral oil, 25%
Kolantyl (Merrell-National)	a. Gel b. Tab. c. Wafer	a. 150 mg b. 300 mg c. 180 mg	X	a. 150 mg b. 185 mg c. 170 mg	X
Krem (Mallinckrodt)	Tab.	X	400 mg	X	Magnesium carbonate, 200 mg; Milk solids, 500 mg
Kudrox (Kremers-Urban)	a. Tab. b. Liq.	a. 400 mg b. 565 mg/tsp	X	a. X b. 180 mg/tsp	a. (S) b. (S)
Maalox (Rorer)	Liq.	225 mg/tsp	X	200 mg/tsp	(S)
Maalox No. 1 & No. 2 (Rorer)	Tab.	#1. 200 mg #2. 400 mg	X	#1. 200 mg #2. 400 mg	(S) (S)
Mylanta (ICI)	Tab. Liq.	200 mg/tab or tsp	X	200 mg/tab or tsp	Simethicone, 20 mg/tab or tsp; (S)

Brand (Manufacturer)	Delivery Form	Aluminum Hydroxide	Calcium Carbonate	Magnesium Oxide, Hydroxide, or Trisilicate	Other Active Ingredients[2]
Mylanta II (ICI)	Tab. Liq.	400 mg/tab or tsp	X	400 mg/tab or tsp	Simethicone, 30 mg/tab or tsp; (S)
Phillips' Milk of Magnesia (Glenbrook)	a. Tab. b. Liq.	X	X	a. 311 mg b. 450 mg/tsp	X
Ratio (Warren-Teed)	Tab.	X	400 mg	X	Magnesium carbonate, 50 mg; (S)
Riopan (Ayerst)	Tab. Chew. Tab. Liq.	X	X	X	Magaldrate, 400 mg/tab or tsp
Robalate (Robins)	Tab.	X	X	X	Dihydroxyaluminum aminoacetate, 525 mg
Rolaids (Warner-Lambert)	Tab.	X	X	X	Dihydroxyaluminum, 324 mg; (S)
Titralac (Riker)	a. Tab. b. Liq.	X	a. 420 mg b. 1000 mg/tsp	X	a. Aminoacetic acid, 180 mg b. Aminoacetic acid, 300 mg/tsp (S)
Tums (Lewis/Howe)	Tab.	X	500 mg	X	X

1. In the form of magnesium trisilicate
2. (S) indicates that caution is required if on a salt-restricted diet.

Constipation

GENERAL CONSIDERATIONS

Regularity of Bowel Movements

The widespread notion that a daily bowel movement is necessary for good health is nonsense. If you are healthy, defecation can normally occur anywhere from three times per day to three times per week. The use of laxatives to promote daily bowel movements, when natural body rhythms do not require them, is not natural, may lead to laxative dependence, and can seriously impair normal bowel function.

Constipation and the Use of Laxatives

There are few valid reasons for self-medication with a laxative. Most episodes of constipation are self-limiting and cure themselves with or without medication. Most can be prevented. If you regularly eat fiber or roughage in the form of fruits, vegetables, and whole-grain foods, you not only promote consistent bowel habits but may help prevent such serious disorders as diverticulitis, the irritable bowel syndrome, and cancer of the colon. Drinking enough liquid, getting sufficient exercise, and responding immediately to the evacuative urge will also help prevent constipation.

Because such measures may be impractical if you are elderly,[1] bedridden, run down, or if you must avoid evacuative strain (cardiac or hernia patients), you may need assistance in maintaining adequate bowel habits. Under such circumstances you should consult your doctor.

There may be serious underlying causes if you have chronic difficulty with the frequency or nature of defecation, e.g., the painful production of hard, dry stools. Such conditions require professional attention. Although early overemphasis on toilet training, improper diet, and/or irregular bowel habits may lead to chronic constipation, the possibility of serious organic disease makes continuous treatment with laxatives unwise. It may result in severe hemorrhoids, anal fissures, or the depletion of essential body salts. It may mask more serious disease.

If you have isolated episodes of constipation as a temporary change in your usual bowel habits, then self-medication with a laxative agent may be reasonable for short periods of time (not more than 7 days) and at recommended dosage levels. You can treat yourself if the onset of

---

1. A weakened defecating reflex may cause retention of dried or impacted stools.

symptoms has been recent and uncomplicated, and can be related to transient stress, traveling, inactivity, or changes in your diet. If nausea, vomiting, or abdominal pain accompany your constipation, they may indicate incipient or acute appendicitis, which can be severely aggravated by laxative use. Consult your doctor in such cases or in any others complicated by symptoms other than relative infrequency of or difficulty in evacuation. You need similar advice and supervision if drugs may be causing your constipation. Non-prescription antacids and prescription narcotics, antispasmodics, tranquilizers, and antianxiety medications can interfere with normal bowel movements. Hemorrhoids and related irritations of the anus or rectum can lead to suppression of the defecatory urge. Under such circumstances both the primary condition and the secondary constipation should have your doctor's attention.

Laxative Agents

Various classes of active laxative agents are available in non-prescription products. They differ principally in their mode of action.

Bulk-Forming Agents   These are among the safest of laxatives. They promote bowel movement by adding water content and volume to stools and usually result in increased frequency of movement and softening of fecal matter. *You must drink a full 8-ounce glass of water or other fluid* with each dose to prevent possible obstruction of the digestive tract. Evacuation normally occurs within 12–72 hours.

Stimulant Agents   These laxatives increase the frequency of bowel movements by irritating the intestinal lining. If you use these agents for too long, you may become dependent upon them and become chronically constipated. Use products containing these ingredients for no more than 7 consecutive days unless your doctor tells you otherwise. Evacuation generally occurs within 6–12 hours.

Saline Agents   Magnesium and phosphate salts retain water in the intestines, helping to form soft stools. Long-term use of these salts is dangerous, and you should limit self-medication to a maximum of 7 days. If you suffer from a kidney disease (gout, stones, urinary retention, edema, etc.), do not use these agents unless your doctor advises you to. Evacuation generally occurs within 3 hours with oral forms and within 15 minutes with rectal forms.

Stool-Softening Agents   These laxatives increase the absorption of fluids by fecal material. This softening effect may be desirable when stools are hard and dry, when inflammation of the anus or rectum makes evacuation painful, or when you should avoid straining (after surgery, with hernia or heart conditions). Evacuation usually occurs within 12–72 hours with oral forms and within 15 minutes with rectal forms.

Lubricant Agents   Mineral oil and mineral oil emulsion promote more frequent bowel evacuation by slowing water absorption from the intestine. The oil also softens stools and makes their release easier. A doctor's supervision is required if you are treating children under 6, or are run down, pregnant, have difficulty in swallowing, or have abdominal pain. Don't use these products for more than 7 consecutive days. Combinations of mineral oil and stool-softening laxatives are hazardous. Evacuation normally occurs within 6–8 hours.

Combinations of Agents   The combination of no more than 2 different classes of laxatives may be reasonable. You may need a product containing a stimulant ingredient and a stool-softening ingredient if bowel movements are infrequent and if the stools they produce are hard, dry, and painful to release. (See the Self-Treatment Section.)

Rectal Agents   It is generally agreed that an ideal laxative should be non-irritating and nontoxic, exercising its effect only in the lower digestive tract, producing desired evacuation in a few hours, and then ceasing to function altogether. Although no such agent is known, you may find the closest approximation in simple suppository laxatives or enemas which disturb only a short segment of the rectum and colon rather than all 25 feet of a typical digestive tract.

Laxatives and Children

Although most laxatives are safe and effective for children, treatment without a doctor's advice and supervision should be undertaken with caution. Among infants and young children, infrequent evacuation may result from serious bowel abnormalities that require a pediatrician's attention. Try not to show too much concern about your child's bowel habits, as this can produce severe emotional disturbances. Avoid medications that may produce laxative dependence or serious side effects. You should probably consult your doctor in any instance of known or suspected constipation in a child under 12.

SELF-TREATMENT

Self-Treatment with a Laxative May Be Reasonable if—

- your symptoms involve the infrequent or difficult release of stools.

- your constipation occurs as a temporary change in your usual bowel habits.
- your constipation began recently and can be related to temporary stress, traveling, inactivity, or dietary alteration.
- your symptoms are not complicated by nausea, vomiting, or abdominal pain.
- you limit self-medication to a maximum of 7 days.
- the frequency of your bowel movements does not fall within the normal range (3 times/day–3 times/week) over a short period of time.
- the frequency of your bowel movements is normal but the stools they produce are dry, hard, and/or painful to release.

Self-Treatment with a Laxative Is Probably Not Wise if—

- your symptoms are chronic.
- you have been using laxative products regularly.
- your symptoms include nausea, vomiting, or abdominal pain.
- any alteration in your bowel habits persists for more than 2 weeks.
- self-medication produces no effect within 7 days.
- you have been taking such constipating drugs as aluminum- or calcium-containing antacids; pain-killers containing codeine, opium, or morphine; antianxiety drugs (e.g., Elavil, Equanil, or Tofranil); tranquilizers (e.g., Mellaril, Meprobamate, or Thorazine), or antispasmodics (e.g., Combid, Donnatal, or Pro-Banthine).
- you are suffering from painful hemorrhoids or other anal or rectal irritation.

These contraindications to the use of a laxative product are serious enough to require consultation with your doctor.

Before Using a Laxative Product, Consider the Possible Causes of Your Constipation

- Have you become overly dependent on laxative products?
- Have you been less physically active than usual?
- Have you been taking any medications that may interfere with normal bowel movements?
- Have there been alterations in the timing of normal bowel movements because of stress, travel, or changes in eating habits?
- Have your bowel movements simply been less frequent or are they complicated by hard, dry stools that cause discomfort?

- Have you been depressed or experienced other changes in general mood?
- Have you been consuming unusual amounts of such stool-hardening foods as processed cheeses or other dairy products?
- Have you attempted to promote natural bowel movements by increasing the amount of fiber or roughage in your diet (fruits, vegetables, whole grain foods, etc.), by increasing your fluid intake, or by immediately responding to the defecatory urge when it occurs?

How to Select or Evaluate a Laxative Product[1]

It is generally wise—

- to choose products with no more than 2 active laxative ingredients.
- to choose only those products with active ingredients clearly labeled both by name and concentration.
- to choose only those products whose active ingredients are judged safe and effective (see below).

Laxative Ingredients Generally Judged both Safe and Effective[2]

Bulk-Forming Laxatives *Drink a full 8-ounce glass of water or other fluid with each dose* to prevent possible obstruction in the digestive tract.

Cellulose derivatives (carboxymethylcellulose, hemicellulose, and methylcellulose—do not use while taking aspirin or prescription drugs), Dietary Bran, Karaya, Malt Soup Extract, Polycarbophil, and Psyllium preparations (plantago and psyllium derivatives).

Stimulant Laxatives The chronic use of these agents often results in laxative dependence and is a major cause of constipation. Use products containing these ingredients only occasionally and for no more than 7 days.

---

1. Based on recommendations of the FDA Advisory Review Panel on Over-the-Counter (OTC) Laxative, Antidiarrheal, Emetic, and Antiemetic Drug Products as published in the *Federal Register,* March 21, 1975
2. Consult your pharmacist about the dosage strength appropriate for you.

> Anthraquinones (may discolor the urine): Cascara Sagrada (bark, casanthranol, extract, and fluidextract), Danthron, Senna, and Sennosides.
>
> Bisacodyl (may produce cramping, rectal burning, faintness, and/or abdominal discomfort).
>
> Castor Oil (may cause excessive loss of water and essential salts; use no more than 1 dose for each infrequent episode of constipation).
>
> Dehydrocholic Acid (not for use in children under 12).
>
> Phenolphthalein (may color urine or stools pink; cease medication if a skin rash appears).

Saline Laxatives   Chronic use of these salts is dangerous and self-medication should be limited to a maximum of 7 days. If you suffer from a kidney disease (gout, stones, urinary retention, hypertension or edema), don't use these agents unless your doctor recommends them.

> Magnesium (citrate, hydroxide, and sulfate); Disodium Phosphate (Oral/Rectal); Monosodium Phosphate (Oral/Rectal); Sodium Biphosphate (Oral/Rectal); and Sodium Phosphate (Oral/Rectal).

Water-Retaining Laxatives   (Suppositories/Enemas)

> Glycerin (may cause rectal itching, burning or slight bleeding), Sorbitol.

Stool-Softening Laxatives   Use these agents when stools are dry and hard, when evacuation is painful because of inflammation of the anus or rectum, or when straining is unwise (after surgery, with hernia or heart conditions, etc.).

> Dioctyl Calcium Sulfosuccinate (DCS), Dioctyl Potassium Sulfosuccinate (DPS), and Dioctyl Sodium Sulfosuccinate (DSS).

Lubricant Laxatives   Use of mineral oil and mineral oil emulsion for children under 6 years of age, or if you are run down, pregnant, have difficulty in swallowing, or have abdominal pain, requires your doctor's supervision. Self-treatment should last no more than 7 consecutive days. Combining mineral oil and stool-softening laxatives is hazardous.

> Mineral Oil (use in oral or rectal form only at bedtime) and Mineral Oil Emulsion (use orally on arising and at bedtime).

Carbon Dioxide Laxatives Combinations of sodium biphosphate, sodium bicarbonate, and sodium acid phosphate in suppository form release carbon dioxide (gas) in the rectum. The resulting pressure may lead to evacuation of the bowels.

Laxative and Non-Laxative Ingredients Generally Judged Unsafe or Ineffective

Belladonna alkaloids, bismuth subnitrate, calomel (mercuric chloride), capsicum, caroid papain, carrageenan (degraded), colocynth, elaterin, gamboge, ginger, ipecac, ipomea, jalap, minerals, multivitamin preparations, podophyllum, and thiamin.

It is probably wise to avoid products containing any of these ingredients.

Laxative Ingredients Whose Safety, Effectiveness, or Appropriate Dosage Strength Is Uncertain

Agar, aloin, bile salts, bran tablets, calcium pantothenate, native carrageenan (Chondrus crispus), Chinese rhubarb, frangula, guar gum, poloxalkal (Polykol), prune concentrate and powder, sodium oleate, tartaric acid, and tartrate compounds.

Fixed-Combination Laxative Products

Combinations of laxative ingredients should contain no more than 2 of the agents previously described as both safe and effective. Consult your pharmacist about the right dosage and combination for you.

PRODUCT CHART

A Selected List of Laxatives

Brand (Manufacturer)	Delivery Form	Mode of Action			Other Laxative Ingredients
		Bulk Former	Lubricant/Softener[1]	Stimulant[2]	
Alophen (Parke-Davis)	Tab.	X	X	Aloin, 16.2 mg; Phenolphthalein, 32.3 mg	Belladonna, 2.7 mg; Ipecac, 4.32 mg
Black-Draught (Chattem)	a. Powder b. Tablet c. Syrup	X	X	Senna: a. 660 mg/g b. 300 mg c. 175 mg/ml	X
Caroid and Bile Salts (Sterling)	Tab.	X	X	C. sagrada extract, 48.6 mg; Phenolphthalein, 32.4 mg	Bile salts, 70 mg; Capsicum, 6 mg; Caroid, 75 mg
Carter's Little Pills (Carter)	Tab.	X	X	Aloe, 16 mg; Podophyllum, 4 mg	X
Casakol (Upjohn)	Cap.	X	Polykol, 250 mg.	Casanthranol, 30 mg	X
Cas-Evac (Parke-Davis)	Liq.	X	X	C. sagrada, 200 mg/100 ml	X
Correctol (Plough)	Tab.	X	DSS, 100 mg	Phenolphthalein, 64.8 mg	X
Dialose (ICI)	Cap.	Carboxymethylcellulose, 400 mg	DSS, 100 mg	X	X

	Form	Carboxymethylcellulose, 400 mg	DSS, 100 mg	Casanthranol, 30 mg	
Dialose Plus (ICI)	Cap.				X
Dorbane (Riker)	Tab.	X	X	Danthron, 75 mg	X
Dorbantyl (Riker)	Cap.	X	DSS, 50 mg	Danthron, 25 mg	X
Dorbantyl Forte (Riker)	Cap.	X	DSS, 100 mg	Danthron, 50 mg	X
Doxan (Hoechst-Roussel)	Tab.	X	DSS, 60 mg	Danthron, 50 mg	X
Doxidan (Hoechst-Roussel)	Cap.	X	DSS, 60 mg	Danthron, 50 mg	X
Doxinate (Hoechst-Roussel)	a. Yellow Cap. b. Green Cap.	X	a. DSS, 240 mg b. DSS, 60 mg	X	X
Dr. Caldwell's Senna Laxative (Sterling)	Liq.	X	X	Senna extract, 412 mg/tsp	X
Dulcolax (B-I)	a. Tab. b. Suppos.	X	X	a. Bisacodyl, 5 mg b. Bisacodyl, 10 mg	X
Effersyllium (ICI)	Powder	Psyllium colloid, 3 g/1½ tsp	X	X	X
Ex-Lax (Ex-Lax)	a. Tab. b. Choc. Tab. c. Powder	X	X	a. Phenolphthalein, 97.2 mg b. Phenolphthalein, 97.2 mg c. Phenolphthalein, 100 mg/pkt	X

Brand (Manufacturer)	Delivery Form	Mode of Action			Other Laxative Ingredients
		Bulk Former	Lubricant/Softener[1]	Stimulant[2]	
Feen-A-Mint (Plough)	Gum Tab.	X	X	Phenolphthalein, 97.2 mg Phenolphthalein,	X
Fleet Enema (Fleet)	Enema	X	X	X	Sodium biphosphate, 16 g/100 ml; Sodium phosphate, 8 g/100 ml
Fleet Pediatric Enema (Fleet)	Enema	X	X	X	Sodium biphosphate, 16 g/100 ml; Sodium phosphate, 6 g/100 ml
Fletcher's Castoria (Glenbrook)	Liq.	X	X	Senna, 6.5%	X
Gentlax (Purdue-Frederick)	Tab. Granules	Guar gum, 1 g/tab. or tsp	X	Senna, 326 mg/tab. or tsp	X
Haley's M-O (Sterling)	Liq.	X	Mineral oil, 25%		Milk of Magnesia, 75%
Hydrolose (Upjohn)	Syrup	Methylcellulose, 5.91 g/2 tbl	X	X	X
Maltsupex (Abbott)	Tab.	Malt soup extract	X	X	X
Metamucil (Searle)	Powder	Psyllium mucilloid, 50%; Hemicellulose, 50%	X	X	X

Product (Manufacturer)	Form	Ingredients		
Mucilose (Winthrop)	Flakes, Powder, Granules	Psyllium, 50%; Hemicellulose, 50%	X	X
Nature's Remedy (Lewis-Howe)	Tab.	Aloe, 143 mg; C. sagrada, 127 mg	X	X
Petro-Syllium No. 1 (Whitehall)	Liq.	Mineral oil, 47.5 g/100 g	Psyllium seed, 750 mg/100 g	X	X
Phillips' Milk of Magnesia (Glenbrook)	Tab., Liq.	See Antacid Product Chart	X	X
Rectalad (Denver)	Enema	Glycerin, 76%; Soap, 5%	DPS, 5%	X	X
Sal Hepatica[3] (Bristol-Myers)	Granules	Sodium carbonate, citrates, phosphate; Citric acid	X	X
Saraka (Plough)	Granules	Karaya gum	Frangula	X	X
Senokot (Purdue Frederick)	a. Gran. b. Tab. c. Suppos. d. Syrup	Senna conc.: a. 326 mg/tsp b. 187 mg c. 652 mg d. 218 mg/tsp	X	X
Serutan (Williams)	Powder, Granules	Psyllium, 100%	X	X

1. Dioctyl Sodium Sulfosuccinate (DSS); Dioctyl Potassium Sulfosuccinate (DPS)
2. Cascara (C)
3. Not for use with a salt-restricted diet

Diarrhea

GENERAL CONSIDERATIONS

Diarrhea, the frequent release of loose or watery stools, is a symptom rather than a disease. It is associated with at least 50 different disorders or conditions whose severity ranges from the relatively mild and transient to the serious and chronic. Acute episodes may result from anxiety or tension; bacterial, viral, or parasitic infection; various prescription and non-prescription drugs; intestinal irritations; malignancies; and/or food poisoning. Chronic or frequent diarrhea may result from continuous emotional distress; intestinal surgery; bowel ulcerations; inherited intolerance of dairy products; parasites; hormonal imbalance; and/or intestinal abnormalities. Whatever its ultimate cause, the immediate symptom results from excess water that remains in your intestines during digestion. Treatment involves capturing excess fluid with water-attracting compounds (adsorbents) or slowing the passage of digestive fluid through the intestinal tract so that normal water reabsorption can occur.

You can probably treat isolated incidents of diarrhea safely yourself if you don't have severe symptoms or complicating health factors. While varying degrees of nausea, vomiting, abdominal cramping, or loss of appetite are not uncommon, if you have a high fever (100° F. or more) or black, tarry stools, you need immediate medical attention. Consult your pediatrician before treating children under 3, because losing too much water can easily be fatal to infants. Excessive dehydration poses a similar threat to pregnant women, who should consult their obstetrician without delay. Because diarrhea weakens you, if you are over 60; experience repeated attacks; or are already run down by such chronic illnesses as asthma, ulcers, heart disease, or kidney disorders, you should seek medical assistance. The mild and temporary diarrhea for which self-treatment is safe is self-limiting and generally disappears within 48 hours, whether or not medication is used. Because the symptom may indicate serious disease, see your doctor if your diarrhea lasts more than 2 days.

Self-Treatment

Because diarrhea may result from many different causes, its origin is often difficult to establish. However, a simple review of possible causes may assist you, your pharmacist, or your doctor in selecting an appropriate treatment. Antibiotics, magnesium-containing antacids, large doses of vitamin C, laxatives, or other medications may cause a bout of diarrhea. Unusual tension, travel, or a diet with fatty or spicy foods, excessive roughage, or foods you do not tolerate well may cause changes in the digestive tract leading to loose and watery stools. Poisoning may come from foods tainted with ameba or other parasites, bacterial toxins, or viruses. In such instances all those who have shared a meal may have severe stomachache, loss of appetite, muscular ache, and fever as well as diarrhea. Episodes of loose and watery stools may follow your use of an enema or other laxative agent.

You can treat diarrhea yourself if your symptoms are mild to moderate, have had a rapid onset, and are not complicated by factors of extremes in age, physical weakness, or chronic disease. Avoid solid foods and drink only such liquids as clear soups or fruit juices. Increase your fluid intake to compensate for water loss, and get adequate rest.

Non-prescription medications can only alleviate symptoms. They do not affect the causes of diarrhea.

Opium as a powder or tincture (liquid), as morphine (an opium derivative) or as paregoric slows the passage of liquids through the intestines so that more water is reabsorbed and more solid stools are formed. Although opium is addictive, the amounts available in non-prescription products are generally safe when used as directed. Products containing opium in any form are available only by prescription in some states. Where it is available, concentrations are often too low to give relief.

Adsorbents (kaolin, pectin, attapulgite, activated charcoal) are commonly included and available in antidiarrheal products. Water, bacteria, viruses, poisons, and other contents of the intestines may cling to these compounds so that less-fluid stools may form. Adsorbents are generally available in liquid or suspension. They are taken after each bowel movement until you achieve control. Although these agents are safe in recommended doses, their effectiveness is not entirely proved.

Astringents (alumina powder, bismuth salts, calcium hydroxide, phenyl salicylate, and zinc phenolsulfonate) are claimed to cause the solidification of protein in the bowels, thereby helping to form less watery stools. Although these agents are safe in recommended doses, there is little available evidence for their effectiveness.

A number of antacids (alumina, calcium carbonate, and other calcium compounds) may prove constipating when taken for the relief of heartburn or acid indigestion. Because the causes of excessive stomach acidity and diarrhea are generally different, whether this constipating side effect will occur when you have diarrhea is questionable.

Anticholinergics (atropine and belladonna alkaloids) slow the passage of digestive fluids through the intestines. However, effective concentrations are not available in non-prescription medications.

Lactobacillus *preparations* The flushing action of diarrhea upsets the normal bacterial population of the bowels. Such bacteria as *Lactobacillus acidophilus* or *Lactobacillus bulgaricus* may help restore this balance. Although safe for use at recommended dosages, the effectiveness of such medication is not proved.

Warning: A number of antidiarrheal products contain amounts of sodium, potassium, or magnesium that may be harmful if you are following a salt-restricted diet or suffer from kidney diseases. Precautionary warnings are included on the label. Observe them with care.

SELF-TREATMENT

Self-Treatment with an Antidiarrheal Product May Be Reasonable if—

- your principal symptom is the unusually frequent release of watery stools.
- your diarrhea is accompanied only by varying degrees of abdominal cramping, nausea, vomiting, or loss of appetite.
- the onset of your symptoms has been rapid and without prior warning of illness.
- you limit self-treatment to a maximum of 48 hours.

Self-Treatment with an Antidiarrheal Product Is Probably Unwise if—

- your symptoms include a fever of more than 100° F.
- your symptoms include bloody, black, or tarry stools.
- you are treating a child younger than 3.
- you are more than 60.
- your symptoms last more than 48 hours.
- you suffer from any chronic or acute disease.
- there have been notable changes in bowel habits prior to the onset of diarrhea.
- you have been taking such prescription medications as tetracycline, lincomycin, ampicillin, erythromycin, clindamycin, neomycin, reserpine, guanethidine, or any antihypertensive drugs.
- you are pregnant.
- you are weakened or run down (possibly by such chronic illnesses as asthma, ulcers, heart disease, diabetes, or kidney disorder).
- you suffer from frequent or long-lasting episodes of diarrhea (particularly if accompanied by loss of appetite or weight, or by general weakness).

These complicating factors are important—see your doctor immediately.

Before Selecting a Non-Prescription Antidiarrheal, Consider the Possible Sources of Your Discomfort

- Have you been suffering from unusual tension, stress, or anxiety?
- Have you been or are you now traveling?
- Have you recently consumed fatty or spicy foods, abnormal amounts of roughage, or foods which generally disagree with you?
- Have you been taking prescription drugs or large doses of non-prescription vitamin C (ascorbic acid), magnesium compounds (milk of magnesia, antacids, or buffered aspirin), enemas, or laxatives?
- Have you been dining with others who are also experiencing similar symptoms?
- Has the onset of your diarrhea been rapid or has your condition been more or less chronic?

Your answers to these questions are important to you, to the pharmacist who will help you select a non-prescription antidiarrheal, and/or to the doctor you may have to consult.

Self-Treatment of Diarrhea

- If your symptoms seem appropriate for self-medication, select a product according to the criteria below, with the assistance of your pharmacist.
- If you have not gained control of your symptoms within 24 hours, consult your pharmacist again. After 48 hours without adequate relief, consult your doctor.
- During self-treatment be certain to rest, drink plenty of liquids (to combat dehydration), consume only liquid nourishment (clear soups and juices), and avoid alcohol, caffeine, and tobacco as much as possible.

How to Select or Evaluate a Non-Prescription Antidiarrheal Product[1]

In general, it is wise to choose only those products—

- which contain a maximum of 2 medically active antidiarrheal agents. In principle, the fewer the ingredients, the better.

---

1. Based on recommendations of the FDA Advisory Review Panel published in the *Federal Register*, March 21, 1975

- whose medically active ingredients are listed by name and dosage strength.

Medically Active Antidiarrheal Agents Generally Judged Both Safe and Effective in Recommended Dosages[1]

Opium (as a powder or tincture; as morphine; or as paregoric); Polycarbophil.

Opium and its derivatives are potentially addictive and may be obtained only by prescription in some states. Risk of addiction is slight at concentrations found in non-prescription antidiarrheals. Because these compounds depress the central nervous system, they should not be used with alcohol, antihistamines, sedatives, barbiturates, or antianxiety drugs.

Antidiarrheal Agents Generally Judged Safe but of Uncertain Effectiveness in Recommended Dosages[1]

Adsorbents In theory adsorbents bind the excess water of diarrhea along with bacteria, poisons, or viruses that may cause the symptoms. This action may aid in the formation of solid stools. Evidence exists for this effect but is not conclusive.

Attapulgite (aluminum-magnesium silicate); charcoal; kaolin (hydrated aluminum) and pectin are commonly used adsorbents.

Anticholinergics Atropine sulfate, homatropine methylbromide, and hyoscyamine sulfate are generally judged as effective in reducing diarrhea. However, the probable minimum dose needed for relief (.6–1 mg) is not found in any non-prescription product. This minimum dose is *not* safe for self-treatment. Avoiding non-prescription antidiarrheals containing anticholinergic agents is probably wise.

Astringents It is claimed that astringents may help form solid stools by precipitating (making solid) proteins in the intestines. Valid evidence for this claim is lacking.

Alumina powder, bismuth salts (subnitrates and subsalicylates), calcium hydroxide, phenyl salicylate (salol), and zinc phenolsulfonate are commonly used astringents.

Other Agents Some bacteria, bulk-forming compounds, and certain antacids have claimed antidiarrheal activity. These include calcium

---

1. Consult your pharmacist about the dosage appropriate for you.

carbonate, carboxymethylcellulose, and *Lactobacillus acidophilus* and *Lactobacillus bulgaricus.*

NOTES

1. Only opium in the form of a powder or a tincture (liquid), as paregoric, or as morphine is thought safe and effective, and is generally available for the self-treatment of symptomatic diarrhea. Attaining effective dosages may be difficult since most non-prescription products contain less than is necessary to achieve relief.
2. It is wise to avoid products containing 3 or more of the active ingredients listed in the foregoing. The same is true for products containing any active ingredients not listed.

Reasonable combinations of 2 active ingredients include Kaolin and pectin; Tincture of opium and pectin; Attapulgite and pectin; Kaolin and hydrated alumina powder; *Lactobacillus acidophilus* and carboxymethylcellulose; *Lactobacillus acidophilus* and *Lactobacillus bulgaricus.*

---

3. Among active ingredients generally judged safe but of uncertain effectiveness, the adsorbents are more likely to be effective than the alternatives.
4. The fact that an antacid (alumina powder, calcium hydroxide, calcium carbonate, etc.) may produce a constipating side effect in the presence of acid indigestion does not mean it will be effective in treating diarrhea.

Ingredients Generally Judged of Uncertain Safety or Effectiveness

Aminoacetic acid (glycine), potassium carbonate, rhubarb fluidextract, and scopolamine hydrobromide (hyoscine hydrobromide). It is wise to avoid products containing these ingredients.

PRODUCT CHART

A Selected List of Antidiarrheal Medications

Brand (Manufacturer)	Delivery Form	Adsorbents	Opiates	Other Active Ingredients[1]
Bacid (Fisons)	Tab.	X	X	Carboxymethylcellulose, 100 mg (Ad); *Lactobacillus acidophilus* (B)
Cams (Lacto)	Liq.	X	X	*Lactobacillus acidophilus* (B)
DIA-Quel (International)	Liq.	Pectin, 24 mg/tsp	Paregoric, .75 ml/tsp	Homatropine methylbromide, .15 mg/tsp (AC); Alcohol, 10%
Donnagel (Robins)	Liq.	Kaolin, 6 g/2 tbl; Pectin, 143 mg/2 tbl	X	Hyoscyamine sulfate, Atropine sulfate, & Scopolamine hydrobromide, all (AC)
Donnagel-PG (Robins)	Liq.	Kaolin, 6 g/2 tbl; Pectin, 143 mg/2 tbl	Opium powder, 24 mg/2 tbl	Hyoscyamine sulfate, Atropine sulfate, & Scopolamine hydrobromide, all (AC)
Kalpec (Wyeth)	Liq.	Kaolin, 3 g/2 tbl; Pectin, 270 mg/2 tbl	X	X
Kao-Gest (Eneglotaria)	Liq.	Kaolin, 6 g/2 tbl; Pectin, 130 mg/2 tbl	X	X
Kaomagma (Wyeth)	Liq.	Kaolin, 6 g/2 tbl	X	X
Kaopectate (Upjohn)	Liq.	Kaolin, 5.8 g/2 tbl; Pectin, 130 mg/2 tbl	X	X

Lactinex (Hynson, Westcott & Dunning)	Tab. Gran.		X	*Lactobacillus acidophilus* (B); *Lactobacillus bulgaricus* (B)
Parelixir (Purdue Frederick)	Liq.	Pectin, 145 mg/2 tbl	Paregoric, 4.5 ml/2 tbl	Alcohol, 18%
Parepectolin (Rorer)	Liq.	Pectin, 162 mg/2 tbl; Kaolin, 5 g/2 tbl	Paregoric, 3.7 ml/2 tbl	X
Pargel (Parke-Davis)	Liq.	Kaolin, 6 g/2 tbl; Pectin, 130 mg/2 tbl	X	X
Pepto-Bismol (Norwich)	a. Tab. b. Liq.	a. Bismuth subsalicylate b. Bismuth subsalicylate	X	a. Calcium carbonate, 350 mg (AA); Glycine b. X
Polymagma Plain (Wyeth)	Tab.	Attapulgite, 500 mg; Pectin, 45 mg; Alumina, 50 mg	X	X

1. Antacid (AA); Anticholinergic (AC); Potential adsorbent (Ad); Bacterial ingredient (B)

Hemorrhoids

GENERAL CONSIDERATIONS

Hemorrhoids (piles) are anal or rectal veins that have become swollen and/or inflamed. Such irritated blood vessels may remain entirely within the rectum and cause no distress, or they may slip out of the anus as firm projections which are often tender and painful. Discomfort may include itching (pruritus), bleeding, and/or mucous discharge. The causes for such distress are obscure and varied. Constipation along with straining to defecate; frequent diarrhea; the overuse of laxatives or enemas; excessive sitting, standing, or straining to lift heavy objects; pregnancy and childbirth; antibiotic irritation; certain contraceptives (diaphragms); excessive coughing or sneezing; constipating diets; cirrhosis of the liver; abdominal tumors; or poor anal hygiene can cause or worsen hemorrhoidal conditions. Such varied physical factors may be complicated by hereditary or emotional tendencies to anal stress or tension. As a result, the cause of hemorrhoids is usually difficult to identify. There are also serious conditions whose symptoms mimic the swelling, pain, itch, and bleeding of hemorrhoids. They include bacterial infections, fistulas, fissures, polyps, cryptitis, abscesses, and rectal cancers.

Self-Treatment

Because anal or rectal distress can have so many origins, self-diagnosis is risky. Your doctor can better determine the causes of your discomfort and pain with the techniques at his or her disposal. Such rectal examinations are advisable every year if you are over 40. Reliance on nonprescription preparations and failure to seek medical assistance in the presence of hemorrhoidal symptoms can have serious consequences.

Self-treatment of suspected hemorrhoids can be reasonable only if your symptoms are limited to mild itching or pain that lasts no more than 2–3 days. Because uncomplicated external hemorrhoids tend to subside quickly and spontaneously, continuing discomfort indicates a more serious condition requiring professional attention. Warm sitz baths 3–4 times a day, and your avoidance of highly spiced foods, excessive straining at stools, and strenuous exercise help relieve discomfort. A stool softener (see Constipation, this chapter) can ease the pressure of fecal material as it passes inflamed tissue. Ointments containing anesthetics can relieve itch and pain. Other active ingredients (astringents, anticholinergics, skin respiratory factor, antiseptics, vasoconstrictors, and vitamins) and other delivery forms (suppositories or aerosols) are of questionable value.

SELF-TREATMENT

Self-Treatment with an Antihemorrhoidal Product May Be Reasonable if—

- you seek *temporary* relief from the mild to moderate itching (pruritus), burning, pain, or soreness of simple external hemorrhoids.
- your doctor has recently diagnosed your condition as that of uncomplicated hemorrhoids.
- your symptoms have had a rapid and recent onset without any other symptoms of illness.
- you limit self-treatment to a few days and then see a doctor if your symptoms are not relieved.

Self-Treatment with an Antihemorrhoidal Product Is Probably Not Advisable if—

- your hemorrhoids are accompanied by bleeding or a mucous discharge.
- you are or have been taking any antibiotic drugs (particularly tetracycline, ampicillin, or lincomycin).
- you are seeking to cure, heal, or obtain lasting relief from hemorrhoids.
- any itching is severe.
- you suffer from any shortness of breath, dizziness on standing up, faintness, or nausea.
- any ano-rectal pain is continuous or throbbing.
- any discomfort is so great that it affects such ordinary activities as walking, sitting, or lifting.
- at any time you feel pressure within the rectum.
- you have been using antihemorrhoidal products without relief.
- you can sense or observe any protrusion of tissue from the anus which is tender or painful before, during, or after defecation.

Any of these conditions is serious enough to require your doctor's advice and supervision. Symptoms of many severe conditions may be mistaken for those of hemorrhoids. Treatment with non-prescription hemorrhoidal products may mask these disorders and delay needed medical treatment.

Before Beginning Self-Medication, Consider the Possible Causes of Your Discomfort

- Have you been suffering from chronic constipation or diarrhea?
- Have you had to strain in lifting objects, in childbearing, or in defecating?
- Have you been eating heavily spiced foods (particularly those containing curry, pepper, or chili)?
- Have you been undergoing unusual stress or tension?
- Have you been coughing or sneezing with abnormal frequency?
- Have you failed to establish healthy bowel habits with a diet enriched by fiber, with adequate fluid intake, and with regular exercise?
- Have you failed to maintain good anal hygiene?
- Have you been using laxatives, suppositories, or enemas with any frequency?

Your answers to these questions are important in defining the possible causes of your discomfort. They should assist you, your pharmacist, and/or your doctor in selecting an appropriate treatment.

How to Select or Evaluate Antihemorrhoidal Products[1]

In general you are wise to remember—

- that external, not internal, hemorrhoids are the usual source of pain and itch.
- that no non-prescription medication can cure hemorrhoids.
- that non-prescription medications can mask symptoms and delay the diagnosis of more severe conditions.
- that non-prescription medications may make existing hemorrhoids worse or cause allergic reactions.

Claimed Active Ingredients

Surface Anesthetics (benzocaine, dibucaine, diperodon, phenacaine, and pramoxine)   These compounds can temporarily relieve the itch

---

1. Based on the FDA Advisory Review Panel report published in the *Federal Register,* March 21, 1975.

or pain of external hemorrhoids if applied directly to inflamed tissue in sufficient quantities and concentration. Allergic reactions to these agents occur frequently and you should cease medication if you notice itching or redness.

Vasoconstrictors Ephedrine, ephedrine hydrochloride, and phenylephrine hydrochloride limit bleeding from anal capillaries on contact. They have little effect on the bleeding from hemorrhoidal veins.

Antiseptics (benzalkonium chloride, resorcin, phenylmercuric compounds, balsam Peru, boric acid, and menthol) In the low concentrations found in non-prescription products, these agents have little effect on bacteria or parasites. Their use may produce allergic reactions which complicate the basic problem.

Astringents and Anticholinergics (tannic acid, bismuth, or zinc compounds, and belladonna compounds) These agents may reduce tissue swelling on contact, but they don't reach hemorrhoidal veins.

Skin Respiratory Factor and Vitamins Claims have been made for the effectiveness of shark- and cod-liver oils and vitamins A and D in promoting the healing of irritated tissues. There is little evidence to support these claims.

Laxatives Stool softeners and other laxatives may relieve constipation that can irritate hemorrhoids. (See Constipation, this chapter.)

Delivery Forms

Ointments The direct application of active ingredients to sites of external pain, inflammation, and itch can best be achieved with ointments. Internal insertion of ointment applicators is hazardous.

Suppositories Since these are inserted into the anus, they often do not make contact with the external hemorrhoidal veins that cause pain and itch.

Aerosols Delivery of active ingredients to sites of inflammation, pain, or itching is erratic. This delivery form is fastidious but probably ineffective.

PRODUCT CHART

A Selected List of Hemorrhoid Medications

Brand (Manufacturer)	Delivery Form	Anesthetic	Astringent	Lubricant	Other Active Ingredients[1]
A-Caine (AVP)	Oint.	Benzocaine; Diperodon	Bismuth subcarbonate; Zinc oxide	Cod-liver oil	Phenylephrine (V); Pyrilamine (AH)
Americaine (Arnar-Stone)	Oint. Suppos.	Benzocaine	X	Polyethylene	Benzethonium (AS)
Anusol (Warner-Chilcott)	Oint. Suppos.	X	Bismuth subgallate; Zinc oxide	Vegetable oil	Balsam Peru (AS)
Aphco (American)	Oint. Suppos.	Benzocaine	Bismuth salts; Zinc oxide	X	Boric Acid (AS); Balsam Peru (AS)
Calmol 4 (Leeming)	Suppos.	X	Bismuth subgallate; Zinc oxide	Cod-liver oil; Cocoa butter	Balsam Peru (AS)
Diothane (Merrell-National)	Oint.	Diperodon	X	Propylene glycol	Benzoxyquine (AS)
Gentz Wipes (Philips Roxane)	Pad	Pramoxine	Witch hazel	Propylene glycol	Cetylpyridinium (AS)
Hemor-Rid (Columbia)	Oint.	Diperodon	Bismuth subcarbonate; Zinc oxide	Cod-liver oil; Petrolatum	Phenylephrine hydrochloride (V); Pyrilamine (AH)
Lanacane (Combe)	Cream	Benzocaine	Chlorothymol	Water soluble	Phenylmercuric acetate (AS)
Mamol (Abbott)	Oint.	X	Bismuth subnitrate	X	Phenylmercuric acetate (AS)

Manzan (DeWitt)	Suppos.	Benzocaine	Zinc oxide	X	X	Phenylpropanolamine (AH); Phenol (AS)
Nupercainal (Ciba)	Oint.	Dibucaine	X	X	X	
Nupercainal Suppository (Ciba)	Suppos.	Dibucaine	Zinc oxide; Bismuth subgallate	Cocoa butter	X	
Pazo (Bristol-Myers)	a. Oint. b. Suppos.	Benzocaine	Zinc oxide	a. Petrolatum; Lanolin b. Vegetable Oil	Ephedrine sulfate (AC); Camphor (AS)	
Preparation H (Whitehall)	Oint. Suppos.	X	X	Shark-liver oil	Yeast cell extract (SRF); Phenylmercuric nitrate (AS)	
Proctodon (Rowell)	Cream	Diperodon	X	X	X	
Proctofoam (Reed & Carnrick)	Foam	Pramoxine	X	Petrolatum; Mineral oil	X	
Rantex (Holland-Rantos)	Pad	X	Witch hazel	Lanolin	Benzalkonium chloride (AS)	
Tanicaine (Upjohn)	Suppos.	Phenacaine	Zinc oxide; Tannic acid	X	Atropine (AC); Phenol (AS)	
Tucks Cream & Ointment (Fuller)	Cream Oint.	X	Witch hazel	Lanolin; Petrolatum	X	
Tucks Pads (Fuller)	Pad	X	Witch hazel	Glycerin	Benzalkonium chloride (AS)	
Vaseline Hemorr-Aid (Chesebrough-Pond)	Oint.	X	X	Petrolatum	X	

1. Anticholinergic (AC); Antihistamine (AH); Antiseptic (AS); Vasoconstrictor (V); Skin Respiratory Factor (SRF)

Motion Sickness and Stomach Upset

GENERAL CONSIDERATIONS

Nausea and vomiting are symptoms of appendicitis, urinary infections, brain injury, heart disease, and/or digestive tract disorders. The morning sickness of pregnancy and reactions to certain drugs, e.g., antibiotics, steroids, cardiac stimulants, may also upset your stomach. Your doctor must diagnose and treat all of these conditions. Only the nausea and vomiting of motion sickness can be reasonably treated with non-prescription products (antiemetics).

The FDA Advisory Review Panel concerned with antiemetics recognizes 3 medically active ingredients as safe and effective for preventing or easing nausea and vomiting.[1] They are cyclizine, meclizine, and dimenhydrinate. All 3 compounds may produce drowsiness and driving a car or operating machinery is dangerous while under their influence. The simultaneous use of alcohol, tranquilizers, or other sedatives may cause severe physical and emotional depression. Conditions such as glaucoma or an enlarged prostate may get worse with frequent use. Blurred vision and a dry mouth are common side effects. Compounds containing phosphate and a carbohydrate (levulose) produce fewer side effects, but their effectiveness has yet to be proved. Products containing bismuth salts, which are claimed to coat the stomach wall, are probably of little use in preventing or relieving upset.

SELF-TREATMENT

Use of an Antiemetic May Be Reasonable if—

- you suffer from motion sickness and will use an antiemetic as a preventive medication.
- you will consume no alcohol, use no prescription medication, nor operate any machinery while taking the medication.

Consult your pharmacist about proper dosages.

---

1. *Federal Register*, March 25, 1975

Use of an Antiemetic Is Unwise if—

- nausea or vomiting result from anything but motion sickness.
- you or the individual for whom you are responsible is very young or is elderly.
- you are or may be pregnant (even if you ordinarily suffer from motion sickness and usually use an antiemetic with no ill effect).
- you experience vomiting unrelated to motion.

Consult your doctor, particularly if nausea or vomiting occurs more than once or twice.

PRODUCT CHART

A Selected List of Antiemetic Medications

Brand (Manufacturer)	Delivery Form	Antiemetic
Bonine (Pfipharmecs)	Chewable Tab.	Meclizine, 25 mg
Dramamine (Searle)	a. Tab. b. Liq.	a. Dimenhydrinate, 50 mg b. Dimenhydrinate, 15 mg/tsp
Emetrol (Rorer)	Liq.	Dextrose; Levulose; Orthophosphoric acid
Pepto-Bismol (Norwich)	Liq.	Bismuth subsalicylate
Pepto-Bismol Chewable Tab. (Norwich)	Tab.	Bismuth subsalicylate; Calcium carbonate

5
WEIGHT CONTROL

GENERAL CONSIDERATIONS

Weight and Weight Control

To achieve weight loss requires a consistent reduction in energy input relative to energy output. Consuming fewer calories and/or increasing caloric expenditure are the only significant weight-altering possibilities available without medical intervention. Non-prescription products may assist you in controlling food intake. They cannot themselves remove poundage. You may possibly be able to suppress your appetite before meals with caffeine or low-calorie candies that elevate blood sugar levels. Bulk-producing agents which swell up in the digestive tract may create a sense of fullness, which discourages eating. Phenyl-propanolamine, a compound related to the prescription amphetamines, may decrease the desire to eat, but you probably should not use it if you suffer from heart disease, hypertension, hyperthyroidism, or diabetes. Surface anesthetics such as benzocaine may desensitize your taste buds and help control your craving for food. The use of artificial sweeteners is a subject of public controversy; whether saccharin and related substances cause human cancers is presently uncertain. That they do eliminate the calories and the negative side effects of sugar is unquestioned. Whole diet substitutes in nutritionally balanced powder, liquid, soup, or cookie form are meant as calorie-controlled substitutes for usual solid foods. Although available without prescription, their exclusive use requires your doctor's advice and supervision. The inclusion of vitamins and minerals in any weight control product is meant to ensure your getting the recommended daily amounts (RDAs) of these essential compounds and elements while dieting.

Childhood Obesity

Although hereditary glandular malfunction accounts for only a small fraction of problems with obesity, if one or both parents are obese, a child faces a statistical probability of becoming an overweight adult. Family eating habits can not only establish patterns of overeating but may create an actual physical basis for obesity. The number of fat storage cells seems to be established and remain fixed by the time you reach adolescence. An overweight child will develop larger numbers of these cells than children who maintain a normal weight throughout development. Those individuals with larger numbers of fat storage cells seem prone to obesity throughout their lives.

SELF-TREATMENT

Self-Treatment with a Weight Reduction Aid May Be Useful if—

- you are in good health and weight loss is desirable.
- you use medication only to assist in reducing your total caloric intake.

Self-Treatment with a Weight Reduction Aid Is Probably Not Wise if—

- you expect to lose weight through the action of a medication alone.
- you suffer from high blood pressure, nervous tension, heart disease, or kidney disorders.

Before Choosing a Weight Reduction Aid, It Is Wise—

- to consult your doctor (particularly if you must lose large amounts of weight, e.g., 10 pounds or more). The medical profession has various weight reduction techniques and medications which are not available to the general public.
- to remember that weight reduction can only occur by reducing caloric intake or increasing caloric expenditure. Non-prescription medications can at best assist you in limiting your daily consumption of calories.
- to avoid crash diets. If weight loss must be rapid (more than a few pounds per week), you must have medical assistance and supervision.
- to select a diet that provides essential vitamins and minerals.
- to remember that permanent weight loss requires a permanent alteration in eating habits.

Claimed Non-Prescription Aids to Weight Reduction

Appetite Suppressants Phenylpropanolamine hydrochloride is an oral decongestant (see Chapter 2). It causes the constriction of blood vessels (capillaries) throughout the body. A secondary effect is its claimed ability to reduce the desire to eat. Non-prescription weight reducing aids may contain phenylpropanolamine in concentrations ranging from 25 mg to 75 mg per dose. That such concentrations can actually suppress the appetite is unproved. That such concentrations can cause nervousness, increased blood pressure, headache, and nausea is certain. Unless your doctor advises otherwise, it is probably wise to avoid this drug if you suffer from heart disease, diabetes, hypertension, hyper-thyroidism, or glaucoma or if you are currently taking guanethidine, debrisoquin sulfate, bethanidine, or other MAO inhibitor.

Bulk Producers   In theory carboxymethylcellulose, psyllium com-pounds, and methylcellulose will absorb water in the digestive tract and produce a sense of fullness which discourages eating. Because these substances remain in the stomach (the source of hunger pangs) for ap-proximately 30 minutes, any sense of fullness is short-lived. Because these agents are principally used for treating diarrhea, their effect may be constipating. Drink at least 8 ounces of fluid with each dose to avoid blocking the intestinal tract.

Surface (Topical) Anesthetics   Benzocaine can deaden sensory nerve endings on contact. A number of non-prescription products include this anesthetic on the theory that it will desensitize taste buds and reduce the desire for food. Paradoxically, many preparations containing ben-zocaine are delivered by tablets or capsules that bypass possible activity in the mouth.

Low-Calorie Candy and Caffeine   Non-prescription products to be consumed prior to a meal may contain low concentrations of sugar or caffeine. In theory, either substance may raise the blood sugar levels and depress the desire to eat. Concentrations in available products are generally too low to achieve such an effect.

Artificial Sweeteners   Saccharin, aspartame, sorbitol, and mannitol are sweetening agents with little or no caloric content. Their widespread inclusion in dietetic foods is meant to assist diabetics in reducing their sugar intake. Because saccharin can cause bladder cancer in rats, it may be withdrawn from use in foods. It may remain on the market as a non-prescription drug available only from pharmacies.

Complete Dietary Products   Nutritionally balanced powders, liq-uids, soups, or cookies containing essential quantities of proteins, fats, and carbohydrates in controlled caloric quantities are widely available. These products are meant as substitutes for usual solid foods. They may produce bowel irregularities and are intended only for temporary weight reducing diets. Do not use them for more than a few consecutive days without your doctor's supervision.

Vitamin and Mineral Supplements   The American diet ordinarily provides more than recommended daily amounts (RDAs) of essential vitamins and minerals. Inclusion of these compounds in weight reduc-tion aids protects you against vitamin or mineral deficiency in case your diet depletes or fails to provide these elements.

PRODUCT CHARTS

CHART A: A Selected List of Appetite Suppressants for Weight Control

Brand (Manufacturer)	Delivery Form	Bulk Former[1]	Phenylpropanolamine Hydrochloride	Other Active Ingredients[2]
Anorexin (Thompson)	Cap.	CMC, 50 mg	25 mg	Caffeine, 100 mg (S); Multiple vitamins
Appedrine (Thompson)	Tab.	CMC, 50 mg	25 mg	Caffeine, 100 mg (S); Multiple vitamins
Ayds (Campana)	Candy	X	X	Multiple vitamins & minerals; Milk solids (S); Vegetable oils
Dex-A-Diet (O'Connor)	Cap.	CMC, 200 mg	X	Multiple vitamins & minerals
Dex-A-Diet (O'Connor)	Chewable Tab.	X	X	Multiple vitamins; Glucose (S)
Dexatrim (Thompson)	Cap.	X	50 mg	Caffeine, 200 mg (S)
Diet-Aid (Rexall)	Tab.	CMC, 100 mg; Alginic acid, 200 mg	X	Sodium bicarbonate, 70 mg (AA)
Grapefruit Diet Plan with Diadex (O'Connor)	a. Tab. b. Cap.	X	a. 10 mg b. 50 mg	Multiple vitamins
Melozets (Calgon)	Wafer	CMC	X	Sugar (S)
Metamucil (Searle)	Powder	Psyllium mucilloid, 50%	X	Dextrose, 50% (S)
Nature's Diet Plan with Diadex (O'Connor)	Tab.	X	75 mg	Multiple vitamins & minerals
Odrinex (Fox)	Tab.	CMC, 50 mg	25 mg	Caffeine, 50 mg (S)

CHART A: A Selected List of Appetite Suppressants for Weight Control

Brand (Manufacturer)	Delivery Form	Bulk Former[1]	Phenylpropanolamine Hydrochloride	Other Active Ingredients[2]
Prolamine (Thompson)	Cap.	X	35 mg	Caffeine, 140 mg (S)
Reducets (Columbia)	Cap.	CMC, 100 mg	X	Benzocaine, 5 mg (AN); Multiple vitamins & minerals
Slim-Line (Thompson)	Candy	CMC, 45 mg	X	Benzocaine, 8 mg (AN); Food solids (21 calories)
Slim-Mint (Thompson)	Gum	CMC, 45 mg	X	Benzocaine, 8 mg (AN)
Spantrol (North American)	Cap.	CMC, 135 mg	75 mg	Benzocaine, 9 mg (AN); Caffeine, 150 mg (S); Multiple vitamins & mineral
Vita-Slim (Thompson)	Cap.	X	50 mg	Multiple vitamins

1. Carboxymethylcellulose or Methylcellulose (CMC). Refer to Chapter 4 (Constipation) for a discussion of these compounds and psyllium.
2. Stimulant, (S); Anesthetic, (AN); Antacid (AA)

CHART B: A Selected List of Sugar Substitutes

Brand (Manufacturer)	Delivery Form	Saccharin
Ril-Sweet (Plough)	Liq.	3.3%
Sucaryl (Abbott)	a. Tab. b. Liq.	a. 5 mg b. .8%
Sweeta (Squibb)	a. Tab. b. Liq.	a. 15 mg b. 14 mg
Sweet & Slim (United)	Powder	Calcium saccharin, 6.5%
Sweet'N Low (Cumberland)	Powder	40 mg/pkt

6
THE SKIN

Acne

GENERAL CONSIDERATIONS

Common acne (*Acne vulgaris*) affects virtually every American adolescent. Myths about its cause and possible cures are many and varied. Contrary to popular opinion, acne probably does not result from improper diet, sexual abnormality, or emotional disorders. Although such factors may aggravate existing conditions, the apparent cause is an excessive production of normal skin oils (sebum) and fats which block hair follicles (pores) on the face, neck, chest, and shoulders. This overproduction of oils is typical of the hormonal changes involved in growing up, and it generally subsides with maturity. In the typical adolescent, self-treatment is reasonable unless symptoms are unusually severe and threaten to produce permanent scarring or serious infection. The outbreak of acne-like symptoms during pregnancy, menstruation, menopause, or middle age may indicate hormonal imbalances requiring your doctor's attention.

Self-Treatment

Acne comedones (pimples) result when pores become blocked with dead cells and excessive amounts of normal skin oils. Combinations of these dead cells and sebum form a plug that clogs the pores and a whitehead results. It may turn black because of skin pigments or surface dirt. If the plug is large, normal skin bacteria may multiply rapidly and produce a local infection (pustules or cysts). Reddening or inflammation indicates that the body's defense mechanisms are acting to isolate and combat infection.

The systematic removal of excess oil from the skin surface and preventing closure of the pores are the goals of self-treatment. Frequent washing with ordinary soap and water helps minimize the accumulation of oils and keep the pores open. Avoiding cosmetics, skin oils, and excessive sweating reduces the likelihood of plug formation. The effects of chocolate, fried foods, nuts, and cola drinks in aggravating acne conditions are uncertain, but eliminating them from the diet can do little harm. The same is probably true for emotional stress. Frequent shampooing and the avoidance of hair oils evidently help in maintaining a dry skin. Non-prescription medications that irritate the skin and promote the rapid peeling of dead tissue help prevent pore blockage. Use them with care since excessive drying may lead to inflammation, itch, or allergic reactions. Careful exposure to the sun both dries excess oils and provides a desired cosmetic effect through tanning.

SELF-TREATMENT

Self-Treatment with a Skin Medication May Be Appropriate if—

- your acne is mild to moderate in nature.
- you are an adolescent or young adult.
- you use a product in conjunction with regular and careful washing of affected skin areas.

Self-Treatment with a Skin Medication Is Probably Not Advisable if—

- your acne produces large pimples or cysts, or leaves your skin visibly scarred or pock-marked.
- you are over 30 years of age.
- you are pregnant. (Acne in pregnancy needs your doctor's attention.)
- medication produces irritation, inflammation, or a general worsening of your condition.
- you rely solely on medication to reduce the symptoms of acne.

Consultation with a dermatologist is wise if any acne condition is severe. Doctors have prescription medications and techniques for treating acute symptoms.

Before Using a Non-Prescription Medication, Remember—

- that regular cleansing of affected areas with ordinary soap and water three to four times per day is probably the most effective technique for avoiding acne.
- that regular shampooing reduces the oiliness of scalp and hair that encourages acne eruptions.
- that the use of hair oils may promote inflammation.
- that squeezing or pinching irritates and inflames the skin and may produce permanent scarring or spread infection.
- that cosmetics may block the pores and help cause acne.
- that the application of any oil to affected areas is apt to worsen existing conditions.
- that moderate amounts of sunlight are beneficial.
- that few, if any, foods are known to aggravate acne conditions but

the avoidance of chocolate, nuts, or fried foods may be wise.
- that sweating or emotional stress may intensify symptoms.

Active Ingredients in Non-Prescription Medications

Benzoyl peroxide (5–10% concentrations) This agent stimulates the growth of skin cells and promotes shedding of the dead tissue that helps cause acne. Because it is a powerful irritant, benzoyl peroxide may produce reddening, sting, and skin warmth, so it should not be applied to sensitive tissue around the eyes, mouth, or neck. If you are fair-skinned, exercise particular caution in using this compound.

Resorcinol (resorcin) In 1–4% concentrations this compound promotes the peeling of dead skin.

Salicylic Acid In 0.5–3% concentrations this compound promotes the peeling of dead skin. It is often combined with resorcinol.

Sulfur Compounds (colloids, sulfides, and thiosulfates) In 1.5–10% concentrations these agents help to dry and reduce already formed blackheads, whiteheads, and pustules. Paradoxically, they have also been implicated in the formation of new pimples.

Surface (Topical) Antibiotics (benzalkonium chloride, cetylpyridinium chloride, chlorhydroxyquinoline, methylbenzethonium chloride, and phenol) Since the bacteria associated with acne are not located at the skin surface, topical antibiotics have little effect on such microorganisms and are of questionable value in controlling infection.

Medicated Soaps The purpose of regularly washing affected areas is to reduce the amount of skin oils. Soaps containing abrasives (aluminum oxide, pumice, or polyethylene), sulfur, salicylic acid, or resorcinol probably have no greater effectiveness than ordinary soap products, since such compounds are rapidly removed by rinsing.

Fats and Oils Products containing petrolatum, lanolin, and cholesterols should probably be avoided since these substances may further block skin pores.

Delivery Forms

(Cleansers, creams, gels, lotions, medicated pads, and ointments) Because oil-based ointments may plug susceptible pores, it is probably wise to avoid them. The choice among other delivery forms is a matter of convenience and personal preference.

A Selected List of Acne Care Medications

Brand (Manufacturer)	Delivery Form	Drying Agents	Peeling Agents (Keratolytics)	Other Active Ingredients[1]
Acne Aid (Stiefel)	a. Oint. b. Liq.	a. Sulfur, 2.5% b. Sulfur, 10%	a. Resorcinol, 1.25% b. X	a. Chloroxylenol (Ab) b. X
Acnederm (Lannett)	Liq.	Sulfur, 5%	X	Zinc sulfate, 1% (AS); Zinc oxide 10% (AS)
Acne-Dome (Dome)	Cleanser	Sulfur	Salicylic acid	X
Acnomel (Smith Kline & French)	a. Oint. b. Cleanser	a. Sulfur, 8% b. Sulfur, 4%	a. Resorcinol, 2% b. Resorcinol, 1%	X
Alphacene (Doak)	Cleanser	Sulfur	Resorcinol	X
Benoxyl (Stiefel)	Lotion	X	Benzoyl peroxide, 5%	X
Clearasil (Vick)	a. Oint. b. Stick	Sulfur, 8%	a. Resorcinol, 2% b. Resorcinol, 1%	a. Bentonite, 11% (AB) b. Bentonite, 4% (AB)
Cuticura (Purex)	Oint.	Sulfur	X	Oil base; Hydroxyquinoline (Ab)
Exzit (Dome)	Cleanser	Sulfur	Salicylic acid	X
Exzit Creme/Lotion (Dome)	a. Oint. b. Liq.	Sulfur	Resorcinol	X

Product	Form			
Fostex (Westwood)	a. Oint. b. Liq. c. Soap	Sulfur, 2%	Salicylic acid, 2%	X
Fostril (Westwood)	Liq.	Sulfur colloid, 2%	X	X
Komed (Barnes-Hind)	Liq.	Sodium thiosulfate, 8%	Resorcinol, 2%; Salicylic acid, 2%	Alumina (AB)
Microsyn (Syntex)	Liq.	Sodium thiosulfate, 8%	Resorcinol, 2%; Salicylic acid, 2%	Alumina (AB)
Neutrogena (Neutrogena)	Soap	Lauryl sulfate	X	X
Pernox (Westwood)	Cleanser	Sulfur, 2%	Salicylic acid, 1.5%	Polyethylene (AB)
pHisoAc (Winthrop)	Oint.	Sulfur colloid, 6%	Resorcinol, 1.5%	X
pHisoDan (Winthrop)	Shampoo	Sulfur, 5%	Sodium salicylate, .5%	Oil base
Propa-pH (Bio)	Liq.	X	X	Boric acid (As); Oil base
Sastid (Stiefel)	Oint.	Sulfur, 1.6%	Salicylic acid, 1.6%	Aluminum oxide (AB)
Thera-Blem (Noxell)	Oint.	Sulfur, 2%	Resorcinol, 1.5%	Phenol (Ab); Oil base
Therapads (Fuller)	Pad	X	Salicylic acid, 1.5%	X
Transact (Westwood)	Gel	Sulfur, 2%	Laureth-4, 6%	X
Xerac (Person & Covey)	Gel	Sulfur, 4%	X	X

1. Antibacterial (Ab); Abrasive (AB); Antiseptic (As); Astringent (AS)

Athlete's Foot

GENERAL CONSIDERATIONS

Athlete's foot, usually *tinea pedis,* is a fungal infection which affects the warm, moist skin between the toes. In severe cases it may spread widely over the feet, producing intense itching, the cracking and drying of the skin, flaking, oozing, and pus. An infectious condition generally confined to adolescents and adults, it is most often contracted through direct exposure to the damp, moist conditions of locker rooms, swimming pools, and gymnasiums. Neglecting fundamental foot hygiene often promotes susceptibility or aggravates existing infection. Frequent and thorough bathing and drying of your feet, changing your shoes and socks daily, and using.absorbent powders can minimize or prevent infestation. Once infection has occurred, you can treat it yourself if the condition remains localized and your symptoms are no more severe than moderate itch, mild skin peeling, and/or superficial splitting of the skin. Widespread inflammation, a tendency to allergic reactions, involvement of toenails, and/or oozing, swelling, bleeding, or intense itch require your doctor's advice and supervision.

SELF-TREATMENT

Self-Medication May Be Reasonable if—

- your infection is superficial and appeared recently.
- your symptoms include mild to moderate sores and/or dry, scaly skin.
- your symptoms include only moderate itching or burning sensations in the affected areas.
- you limit self-medication to no more than 4 weeks before seeing a doctor, particularly if symptoms intensify.
- you practice good foot hygiene.

Self-Medication May Be Unwise if—

- you suffer from excessive sweating, skin allergies, or chronic disorders, e.g., diabetes.
- your infection spreads around or under a toenail.
- inflammation or swelling spreads beyond the skin between the toes.
- sores are moist and oozing.

- inflamed areas do not respond to self-medication after a period of no more than 14 days.
- you are under a doctor's care and your symptoms began after taking a prescription drug.

Consult your doctor if any of these conditions apply to you.

While Using a Non-Prescription Medication, It Is Wise—

- to follow a simultaneous non-medical regimen which may help control or eliminate your fungal infection. This should include changing your shoes and socks daily, washing and thoroughly drying your entire foot frequently, avoiding activities producing perspiration or sweat, wearing light, open footwear, and avoiding locker rooms and swimming pools where infective fungus may be prevalent.
- to use drying agents, e.g., powders, that may absorb excessive moisture.
- to commit yourself to daily foot hygiene and medication for a period of 2–4 weeks.

Active Ingredients in Non-Prescription Products

Fungicides   Various forms of undecylenic acid, acetic acid, caprylic acid, hydroxyquinoline, resorcinol, tolnaftate and zinc compounds can control, if not eliminate, fungal spores and infections. Among these compounds tolnaftate is probably the most effective.

Keratolytics (skin-peeling agents)   Salicylic and benzoic acids lead to the sloughing-off of external skin layers. Shedding of this skin is important since it is the tissue most often infected by the fungus of athlete's foot.

Other Ingredients   Various alcohols, astringents, surface anesthetics, absorbents, and antibacterial agents are often added to non-prescription products to cool, relieve itch, desensitize, dry, or prevent bacterial infections. Their function is generally of secondary importance.

Delivery Forms

(Creams, liquids, gels, ointments, powders, and sprays) Any oil-based cream or ointment may complicate healing and promote bacterial infection. Powders deliver effective active ingredients with less certainty than liquids, gels, or sprays.

PRODUCT CHART

A Selected List of Medications for Athlete's Foot

Brand (Manufacturer)	Delivery Form	Antifungal Agent	Skin Peeling Agent (Keratolytic)	Other Active Ingredients[1]
Campho-Phenique (Sterling)	a. Liq. b. Powder	a. Phenol, 4+% b. Phenol, 2%	X	Camphor (CI)
Compounded Undecylenic Acid (Various)	Oint.	Undecylenic acid, 5%; Zinc undecylenate, 20%	X	X
Desenex (Pharmacraft)	a. Aerosol b. Oint. c. Powder	Zinc undecylenate, 20%; Undecylenic acid: a., c. 2%; b. 5%	X	X
Foot-Guard (Gillette)	Aerosol Powder	Undecylenic acid; Zinc undecylenate	X	X
Fungacetin (Blair)	Liq. Oint. Powder	Triacetin	X	X
Fungi-Spray (Rand)	Aerosol	Benzethonium chloride	X	Benzocaine (A)
NP 27 Aerosol (Norwich)	Aerosol	Zinc undecylenate	Salicylic acid	Dichloro-phene (As)
Quinsana (Mennen)	Powder	Undecylenic acid; Zinc undecylenate	X	X
Solvex (Scholl)	Aerosol	Undecylenic acid; Zinc undecylenate; Chlorothymol	X	Benzocaine (A); Dichloro-phene (As)
Sopronal (Wyeth)	Liq. Oint. Powder	Zinc & sodium caprylates & proprionates	X	X
Tinactin (Schering)	Aerosol Cream Liq. Powder	Tolnaftate, 1%	X	X
Ting (Pharmacraft)	Oint.	Zinc stearate	Benzoic acid	Boric acid (As); Zinc oxide (AS)

1. Anesthetic (A); Antiseptic (As); Astringent (AS); Counterirritant (CI)

Bunions, Corns, Calluses, and Warts

GENERAL CONSIDERATIONS

Foot Discomfort

Bunions   These painful, swollen, and tender growths tend to form on the big toe. They usually result from pressure created by tight shoes or from abnormal posture. Before you can treat a bunion, you need an accurate diagnosis of its cause; you can then remove the source of the irritation. In some cases bunions must be removed surgically.

Corns/Calluses   Any skin tissue exposed to constant pressure or friction will toughen, thicken, and form hard or soft lumps which may prove painful. Such growths on the feet (corns) commonly result from the pressure of tight footwear or from the friction produced by footwear which is too loose. Poor posture, reduced circulation, or diseases affecting the skeletal system may cause similar irritation. You can treat your corn or callus by eliminating the source of chafing or pressure along with hygienic treatment and medication to reduce its size.

Warts   Warts are caused by a common virus which affects not only the feet but areas of skin on the hands, face, and tissue surrounding the anus. The smooth, skin-colored thickenings typical of this viral infection are actually small skin tumors that may grow with repeated irritation. Enlargement frequently occurs on the soles of the feet (plantar warts). Although they are not usually painful, warts spread easily to the face or hands and may cause embarrassment, particularly among adolescents and young adults who are most prone to infection. Self-treatment requires scrupulous hygiene and keratolytic agents, which cause peeling of the toughened skin. Medication is often unnecessary since warts tend to disappear spontaneously.

SELF-TREATMENT

Self-Treatment of Bunions, Corns, Calluses, or Warts May Be Appropriate if—

- the symptoms of your condition are mild to moderate, do not impede ordinary movement, nor cover widespread areas of the skin.

- you are not suffering from any chronic disease.
- you limit self-medication to no more than 4 weeks and see your doctor if symptoms do not improve within that time.
- your condition started recently.

Self-Treatment Is Probably Not Advisable if—

- any condition is severe enough to affect ordinary movement.
- symptoms are widespread and/or involve bleeding or oozing.
- you are taking prescription medications and/or suffer from circulatory diseases (arthritis, diabetes, heart ailments, kidney disease, phlebitis, etc.).
- self-medication does not produce initial relief within a week.

Any of these conditions requires your doctor's advice and supervision.

Before Beginning Self-Medication for Bunions or Corns, It Is Wise—

- to determine whether excessive pressure or friction results from footwear that is too tight or too loose.
- to determine whether poor posture, excessive sweating, or strenuous exercise may be causing abnormal conditions.
- to determine whether your symptoms may result from new shoes or other recent changes in footwear.
- to try non-medical treatments such as warm foot baths, the gentle removal of dead tissue with pumice or other mild abrasive, and the application of protective ointments or pads.

Active Ingredients in Non-Prescription Products

Keratolytic Agents (salicylic acid, zinc chloride, pantothenic acid, acetic and lactic acids) These compounds cause the peeling of tissue. When applied to the toughened skin of corns, calluses, and warts, they cause it to be shed. This reduces the size of such growths, thereby reducing frictional discomfort. In the case of warts such action may eliminate some of the causative virus. Because these agents act on normal as well as toughened skin, limit application to affected areas. At any sign of irritation, redness, or inflammation of healthy tissue, stop medication.

Lubricants, Local Anesthetics, and Astringents Products which soften toughened skin often include castor oil, petrolatum, or mineral oil. Local anesthetics such as benzocaine, dibucaine, and diperodon may reduce localized pain. Their concentration is generally too low to produce desired relief. Camphor, menthol salicylate, and thymol are astringents which may help peel areas of dead skin and can reduce the discomfort of itching or mild pain.

Pantothenic Acid Compounds These agents promote peeling of dead skin and are usually used for the treatment of warts.

Delivery Forms

(Creams, liquids, lotions, ointments, plasters, and medicated pads) Some delivery forms contain medically active ingredients dispersed through collodion mixtures. These substances form a tough film over affected areas and protect the sensitive tissue. Plasters and pads provide additional cushioning against pressure and friction from normal walking or standing.

PRODUCT CHART

A Selected List of Aids for the Treatment of Bunions, Corns, Calluses, and Warts

Brand (Manufacturer)	Delivery Form	Peeling Agents (Keratolytics)	Lubricants/ Protectants	Other Active Ingredients[1]
Blis-To-Sol Corn and Callus (Chattem)	Liq.	Salicylic acid; Zinc chloride	Collodion	Diperodon (A)
Compound W (Whitehall)	Liq.	Salicylic acid; Acetic acid	X	X
Derma-Soft Creme (Creighton)	Oint.	Salicylic acid	Oil base	X
Dr. Scholl's Corn/ Callous (Scholl)	Oint.	Salicylic acid	Oil base	X
Dr. Scholl's (Scholl)	Pads Plasters	Salicylic acid	Protective pads	X
Freezone (Whitehall)	Liq.	Salicylic acid; Zinc chloride	Balsam oil; Collodion	X
Mosco (Corns) Ointment (Moss)	Oint.	Salicylic acid	X	Methyl salicylate (AS)
Quick Aid (Lee)	Liq.	X	Castor oil	X
Wart-X (Hall)	Liq.	Salicylic acid	Castor oil	X

1. Anesthetic, (A); Astringent (AS)

Burns and Sunburns

GENERAL CONSIDERATIONS

Skin tissue is destroyed on contact with flame, scalding liquids, hot objects, caustic chemicals, intense sunlight, electric shock, or X-ray radiation. Damage may range from mild to extensive, with injury to underlying organs, shock, infection, and even death occurring in the most severe instances. The simplest, or *first-degree,* burns affect only the outer layer of skin and produce redness and pain. Burns of the *second degree* penetrate the skin more deeply and produce blisters along with first-degree symptoms. Skin injured by burns of either degree regenerates normally if there is no complicating infection. *Third-degree* burns penetrate the full skin thickness, producing a brown, toughened appearance with little or no blistering. *Fourth-degree* burns reach underlying tissues and organs. They can be recognized by their black, charred appearance, depth, and the presence of severe pain. Skin injured by burns of either the third or fourth degree will not regenerate and grafting is required. Shock, severe infection, and permanent disfigurement can result from these burns.

Self-Treatment

Treat only burns of the first or second degree yourself and then, only if damage does not exceed a few square inches of skin (mild sunburn may be the one exception). Repeated applications of cold, wet compresses help to relieve pain and provide essential fluids to injured tissue cells. It is the injured cells, rather than ones that have been destroyed, that cause sensations of pain and discomfort. Cold acts as a natural anesthetic and should be maintained until the pain subsides. Once this has occurred, you may use non-prescription medications as follow-up therapy. Principal ingredients in burn preparations include surface anesthetics, which may relieve lingering pain, and antibacterial compounds, which may help prevent infection.

Sunburn

Most people treat sunburn far too casually. Although such burns are generally limited to the first or second degree, injury often involves most of the skin and may produce fever, dehydration, shock, and even death. Treat your sunburn with the same care as you would treat burns from other sources. Apply cold, wet compresses to all injured tissue, drink plenty of fluids, and use aspirin or an aspirin substitute (see Chapter 1) if headache develops. It is probably wise to apply non-prescription medications only after pain and skin warmth subside. Consult your doctor immediately if any symptom seems severe.

Severe Burns

Any severe burn requires prompt professional attention. However, immediate first aid can do much to minimize damage before medical assistance arrives. Extinguishing any flame is critical. Gently flooding an injured area with cold water will reduce damage caused by scalding liquids or harsh chemicals while cooling inflamed tissue. The subsequent application of cold, moist compresses may be advisable if the skin is not charred or blackened. Immediate transport to the nearest hospital emergency room, preferably one with a burn care unit, is absolutely essential.

SELF-TREATMENT

Self-Treatment with a Burn Preparation May Be Reasonable if—

- your burn is superficial and is limited to no more than a few square inches of skin.
- your burn is obviously not deep and is accompanied by no symptoms other than reddening of the affected area, simple blisters, and/or mild to moderate pain.
- you have initially treated your burn with cold water, ice, or cold compresses.

Self-Treatment with a Burn Preparation Is Probably Not Wise if—

- your burn affects more than a few square inches of skin (with the exception of mild sunburn).
- your burn is obviously deep and produces no redness or blisters at the center of the affected area.
- the skin appears leathery, black, or dry rather than red and blistered.
- your burn has been caused by harsh chemicals or electric shock.

In these cases immediately consult your doctor and/or report to the nearest hospital, preferably one with a burn care unit. If in doubt about the degree or extent of any burn, get medical assistance.

Before Beginning Self-Treatment with a Burn Product, It Is Wise—

- to be certain that your burn does not require professional medical attention.
- to treat the affected area with ice water or cold water compresses until pain subsides. Any but the mildest of burns requires emergency medical attention to minimize tissue damage, infection, and possible shock. The immediate application of ice water or cold water compresses to the affected area can relieve pain and restore essential fluid to injured cells. Hospitals with burn treatment units are the best equipped to handle severe burns.

Claimed Active Ingredients in Burn Products

Surface (Local) Anesthetics Benzocaine, butamben picrate, diperodon hydrochloride, ethyl chloride, phenylphenol, lidocaine, and tetracaine can desensitize nerve endings, thereby minimizing the sensation of pain arising from burns. A 20% concentration is generally necessary to achieve significant relief. In these concentrations, allergic or poisoning reactions may occur. For this reason many non-prescription products contain too little of the active ingredient to give the desired relief. Use of these agents with serious burns can mask severity, complicate the healing process, or interfere with subsequent medical procedures. Anesthetics do nothing to cure a burn.

Antibacterial Agents Such compounds as Bacitracin, benzethonium chloride, chlorobutanol, chlorothymol, chloroxylenol, 8-hydroxyquinoline, neomycin, povidone, tetracycline, and triclosan are included in many products on the theory that any break in the skin increases the possibility of infection. Whether any of these ingredients is present in sufficient concentration to prevent infection is open to question.

Other Ingredients Alcohol, menthol, and aromatic bases may provide a temporary sensation of cooling as they evaporate, but may aggravate a burn by their dehydrating action. Methyl and sodium salicylate, resorcinol, tartaric acid, and zinc oxide may act as counterirritants.

Delivery Forms

(Ointments, creams, lotions, sprays, and aerosols) The direct application of any medication to a burn surface can complicate healing or interfere with medical procedures that may prove necessary. Ointments, lotions, and creams cover most completely, may promote bacterial infection, and are most difficult to remove. Spray and aerosol forms are probably preferable.

PRODUCT CHART

A Selected List of Burn and Sunburn Medications

Brand (Manufacturer)	Delivery Form	Anesthetic	Antibacterial	Other Active Ingredients[1]
Americaine (Arnar-Stone)	a. Oint. b. Spray	Benzocaine, 20%	a. Benzethonium chloride, .1% b. X	X
Bacimycin (Merrell-National)	Oint.	X	Bacitracin; Neomycin	X
Bacitracin (Pharmaderm)	Oint.	X	Bacitracin	X
Bactine (Miles)	Liq.	X	Methylbenzethonium chloride, .5%; Chlorothymol, .1%	
Betadine (Purdue Frederick)	a. Oint. b. Spray	X	a. Povidone, 10% b. Povidone, 5%	X
Bicozene Creme (Creighton)	Oint.	Benzocaine	X	Resorcinol (SP)
Borofax (Burroughs)	Oint.	X	Boric acid	Lanolin (P)
Butesin Picrate (Abbott)	Oint.	Butamben picrate, 1%	X	X
Desitin (Pfizer)	Oint.	X	X	Various oils (P); Vitamins A & D; Zinc oxide (AS)
Foille (Carbisulphol)	Liq. Oint. Spray	Benzocaine, 2%	Benzyl alcohol; 8-Hydroxyquinoline	Sulfur (SP)
Neo-Polycin (Dow)	Oint.	X	Bacitracin; Neomycin; Polymyxin	X
Noxzema Medicated (Noxell)	Liq. Oint.	X	Phenol, 4%	Various oils (P)

A Selected List of Burn and Sunburn Medications

Brand (Manufacturer)	Delivery Form	Anesthetic	Antibacterial	Other Active Ingredients[1]
Nupercainal (Ciba)	a. Cream b. Oint. c. Spray	Dibucaine: a. .5% b. 1% c. .25%	X	X
Owens Ointment (Owen)	Oint.	X	X	Various oils (P); Vitamins A & D
Peterson's Ointment (Peterson)	Oint.	Carbolic Acid	X	Tannic acid (AS); Zinc oxide (AS)
Pontocaine (Winthrop)	a. Cream b. Oint.	a. Tetracaine, 1% b. Tetracaine, .5%	X	a. X b. Various oils (P)
Quik-Aid (Lee)	Spray	Benzocaine	Benzyl alcohol	X
Solarcaine (Plough)	a. Cream b. Foam c. Lotion	Benzocaine: a. 1% b. .5% c. .5%	Triclosan	X
Surfacaine (Lilly)	Cream Jelly Oint.	Cyclomethycaine	X	X
Terramycin (Pfizer)	Oint.	X	Oxytetracycline	X
Triple Antibiotic (North American)	Oint.	X	Bacitracin; Neomycin; Polymyxin	X
Xylocaine (Astra)	Oint.	Lidocaine, 2.5%	X	X
Zemo (Plough)	Oint.	X	Triclosan; Boric acid	Zinc oxide (AS); Menthol, Methyl salicylate, & Sodium salicylate, all (CI)

1. Astringent (AS); Counterirritant (CI); Protectant (P); Skin Peeling (SP)

Insect Bites and Insect Stings

GENERAL CONSIDERATIONS

Insect Stings

Serious effects or even death may result from some encounters with stinging insects (honeybees, wasps, yellowjackets, bumblebees, and others). Although their poisons are highly toxic, the amounts of injected venom are generally too small to produce more than a localized reaction in most people. However, if you are among that 10% of the general population who are acutely sensitive to even the lowest concentrations of these substances (principally histamine and various amino acids), your reactions may include nausea, vomiting, fainting, breathing difficulties, heart failure, or death. Since sensitivity usually increases after each sting and subsequent reactions are generally more intense, if you are subsequently stung, get emergency medical help at once.

For a majority of those stung by wasps, bees, and similar insects, the venom produces localized pain, swelling, and itch, which may be complicated by scratching and other irritations that lead to secondary bacterial infection. Self-treatment involves the immediate application of ice packs to reduce swelling, removal of the insect stinger, and application of an antiseptic. The subsequent use of non-prescription anesthetics, antihistamines, astringents, and itch-reducing (antipruritic) medications should protect the affected area, reduce irritations, and promote faster healing.

Insect Bites

Ticks, chiggers, mosquitoes, bedbugs, and lice (head, body, or pubic) feed on human blood. They penetrate the skin and may temporarily or more permanently attach themselves to a blood capillary. You know they are there because of the localized reddening, itch, and swelling they cause. Irritations produced by insects that do not permanently attach themselves to the skin, e.g., mosquitoes, generally respond to the kinds of symptomatic relief provided by non-prescription medications. Insects which become firmly attached to the skin may deposit their eggs (nits) within skin layers and may produce chronic discomfort and irritation.[1] Although the discomfort produced by more permanent parasites is rarely severe, it is often annoying. The ingredients in most non-

---

1. In some cases bacterial or viral agents of serious diseases may be introduced into the bloodstream by biting insects (ticks).

prescription medications can provide temporary relief. However, your registered pharmacist and/or doctor can often identify the offending parasite and suggest (or prescribe) medications which will eliminate both the infecting adult and its nits.

SELF-TREATMENT

Self-Treatment with an Insect Bite or Sting Preparation May Be Appropriate if—

- your irritation is localized.
- your symptoms include nothing more serious than mild to moderate redness, itching, swelling, or pain.
- you can identify the offending insect as a bee, wasp, hornet, mosquito, chigger, tick, louse, bedbug, or flea.
- symptoms do not increase following medication.
- you have no previous history of allergy to insect stings or bites, or to skin medications.

Self-Treatment with an Insect Bite or Sting Preparation Is Probably Not Advisable if—

- you have a history of sensitivity to insect bites or stings.
- you suffer from asthma, or have a history of allergic reactions to skin medications, pollens, dust, smoke, etc.
- the origin of your bites or the kind of insect producing them is unknown to you.
- your symptoms are in any way severe.
- you experience excessive sweating, vomiting, shortness of breath, faintness, or feverishness following an insect sting.
- your symptoms are accompanied by fever, chills, headache, or muscle soreness.

These problems require medical attention. Allergic sensitivity to the venom of stinging insects can produce a kind of shock which is frequently fatal. Getting immediate medical attention is critical. Neglecting the complaints of those who seem to exaggerate their reaction to an insect sting has often led to death. If you know you are very allergic to insect venom, you should carry identification indicating the nature of your susceptibility. Carrying an emergency insect-sting kit is wise if you are acutely sensitive.

For Self-Treatment of an Insect Bite or Sting, It Is Wise—

- to apply ice packs to the site of a sting in order to reduce swelling.
- to gently remove the stinger by scraping with a fingernail or other flat object that will not pinch the attached venom sac.
- to identify the possible source of your insect bites. This can help your druggist select a product which may not only relieve symptoms but assist in the destruction of the insect and its eggs.
- to avoid any scratching or other irritation of injured tissue, which can cause inflammation and infection.
- to use non-prescription medications for relieving itch (pruritus), pain or irritation; preventing secondary infection; and protecting wounded tissue.
- to boil all clothing, sheets, and pillow cases if your bites have been caused by bedbugs or lice.

Ingredients Included in Insect Bite and Sting Products

Surface (Local) Anesthetics Benzocaine, dibucaine, tetracaine, and other pain-deadening compounds are included in many non-prescription preparations. Standard concentrations ranging from 1% to 4% are generally insufficient to produce desired relief, particularly since the anesthetic must penetrate skin barriers to reach underlying nerve endings. Such contact may produce allergic reactions, particularly after prolonged use.

Antipruritics/Antihistamines Mild to moderate itching may be relieved by various forms of topical menthol, phenol, or camphor (antipruritics) and various antihistamines (diphenhydramine, methapyrilene, phenyltoloxamine, pyrilamine, or tripelennamine). Reduction in scratching stings and bites is useful in preventing inflammation, bacterial infection, and/or permanent scarring. Prolonged use of antihistamine ingredients may produce allergic reactions.

Astringents Agents such as benzyl benzoate, calamine, resorcin, zinc oxide, and zirconium oxide may protect, dry, and toughen injured skin. Their effectiveness remains unproved. The use of zirconium oxide is questionable since it may produce skin nodules or lumps.

Antibacterials If irritated by scratching or rubbing, the open sores produced by insect stings or bites may become infected. Anti-infective agents such as benzalkonium chloride, benzethonium chloride, hydroxyquinoline, or methylbenzethonium chloride may help prevent such infections. Whether they are present in sufficient concentrations in most non-prescription medications is questionable.

Delivery Forms

(Creams, liquids, lotions, ointments, pads, or sprays) Any oil-based ointment or cream may complicate healing and actually promote secondary infection. Liquids, lotions, and sprays are less likely to produce complications.

PRODUCT CHART

A Selected List of Medications for Insect Bites and Stings

Brand (Manufacturer)	Delivery Form	Anesthetic	Antiseptic/ Antibacterial	Astringent	Counterirritant/ Antipruritic[1]
After-Bite (Tender)	Oint.	X	X	Ammonium hydroxide	Camphor; Various oils
Anti-Itch Cream (Hall)	Cream	Benzocaine; Dibucaine; Tetracaine	X	X	X
Benadryl (Parke-Davis)	Liq.	X	X	X	Benadryl, 2% (AH)
Caladryl (Parke-Davis)	Liq. Oint.	X	X	Calamine	Benadryl (AH); Camphor
Chiggerex (First Texas)	Oint.	Benzocaine	X	X	Camphor; Menthol; Various oils
Chiggertox (First Texas)	Liq.	Benzocaine, 2.1%	Alcohol, 53%	Benzyl benzoate, 21.4%[2]	Soap
Lanacane (Combe)	Oint. Spray	Benzocaine	X	Resorcin[2]	X
Quotane (Smith Kline & French)	Oint.	Dimethisoquin hydrochloride, .5%	X	X	X
Surfadil (Lilly)	Cream Liq.	Cyclomethycaine	X	X	Methapyrilene hydrochloride (AH)
Tucks (Fuller)	Pads	X	Benzylalkonium chloride	X	Glycerin; Methylparaben; Witch hazel

1. Antihistamine ingredient, (AH); an antipruritic relieves itch (pruritus)
2. Skin peeling (keratolytic) agent

Poison Ivy, Oak, Sumac, and Contact Dermatitis

GENERAL CONSIDERATIONS

Poison Ivy, Poison Oak, Poison Sumac, and Contact Dermatitis

Many people are allergic to the oily resin produced by certain plants. Although as many as 75 different varieties of trees, grasses, and shrubs may cause allergic skin reactions, a majority of cases result from direct or indirect exposure to the resins of poison ivy, oak, or sumac (allergens). Symptoms of an allergic reaction usually appear a few hours after contact and typically begin with reddening of the skin and intense itching. Depending on the degree of contact, swollen sores may appear, accompanied by feelings of warmth or burning. Raised blisters often appear over intensely affected areas and tend to leak a watery liquid as they heal. Contrary to general belief, this liquid is not infectious and will not spread inflammation to unaffected skin. However, blisters and their contents need protection since they provide a natural barrier against infection of the injured tissue which lies beneath. If they burst, a secondary infection by airborne micro-organisms may result.

Self-Treatment

Contact with the hair of an animal exposed to poison ivy, oak, or sumac may stimulate an allergic reaction. To avoid repeated contact with the offending allergen, launder all contaminated clothing or animal fur. If you have had no contact with potentially poisonous plant resins, your symptoms may result from sensitivity to various dyes, volatile fluids, lacquers, or glue (contact dermatitis).

If your allergic rash covers large areas or produces very marked swelling, you should consult your doctor immediately. However, if your rash is of a mild to moderate nature, localized to one or a few areas of the body, and produces no more than slightly swollen sores and moderate itching or burning, then self-treatment may be appropriate.

Protection of affected tissues is critical. Reduce the urge to scratch by the careful use of surface antihistamines, menthol, phenol, or camphor. Vigorous washing of affected areas can only make the condition worse. Once sores form you can apply such astringents as aluminum acetate, zinc oxide, or tannic acid to help reduce oozing and inflammation. A similar effect may be achieved by gently bathing affected areas with dressings soaked in sodium bicarbonate or mild salt solutions 3–4 times a day. Nighttime applications of calamine lotion or zinc oxide may continue the desired drying action. If symptoms don't improve, consult your doctor or pharmacist.

SELF-TREATMENT

Self-Treatment of Poison Ivy, Oak, Sumac, or Contact Dermatitis May Be Appropriate if—

- your rash produces sores of a mild to moderate nature.
- your rash is localized to one or a few areas of the body.
- your initial symptoms are limited to redness, slightly swollen sores, itching, and/or burning.
- you can relate the development of your dermatitis to possible exposure to poisonous plants or harsh chemicals.

Self-Treatment of Suspected Poison Ivy, Oak, Sumac or Contact Dermatitis Is Probably Not Advisable if—

- your rash spreads widely over the body.
- your symptoms include fever, considerable swelling, massive blistering, or oozing.
- you are suffering from a chronic disease or are otherwise under a doctor's care.
- you cannot relate the appearance of your symptoms to possible exposure to poisonous plants or harsh chemicals.
- your symptoms get worse following self-treatment.

Severe cases of poison ivy, oak, sumac, or contact dermatitis need a doctor's supervision.

When Beginning Self-Medication, It Is Wise—

- to remember that treatment should protect injured tissue, relieve itching, and hygienically remove the liquid and solid debris which form during healing.
- to keep medication at a minimum. The appearance of skin sores

may provoke you to overmedicate and cause further allergic reactions or secondary infections.

- to avoid the skin irritations produced by frequent bathing, cosmetics, skin lotions, or oily medications.
- to wash any clothing, bedding, or fur which may still contain the poisonous allergen.

Active Ingredients in Non-Prescription Products

The same classes of ingredients used for the treatment of insect stings and bites are found in non-prescription products intended for the treatment of poison ivy, oak, sumac, and contact dermatitis. (See pages 113–114).

Delivery Forms

(Creams, gels, liquids, lotions, ointments, or sprays) Any cream or ointment with an oily base may complicate healing and promote secondary infection. Choice among other forms is a matter of preference and convenience.

PRODUCT CHART

A Selected List of Medications for Poison Ivy, Oak, Sumac, and Contact Dermatitis

Brand (Manufacturer)	Delivery Form	Anesthetic	Antipruritic[1]/ Antihistamine	Antiseptic	Astringent
Anti-Itch Cream (Hall)	Cream	Benzocaine; Dibucaine; Tetracaine	X	X	X
Benadryl (Parke-Davis)	Liq.	X	Benadryl (diphen-hydramine)	X	X
Caladryl (Parke-Davis)	Liq. Oint. Spray	X	Benadryl (diphen-hydramine); Camphor	X	Calamine
Hista-Calma (Rexall)	Liq.	Benzocaine	Phenyl-toloxamine	X	Calamine
Ivy Dry Cream (Ivy)	Cream Liq.	Benzocaine	Camphor; Menthol	X	Tannic acid
Lanacane (Combe)	Oint. Spray	Benzocaine	X	X	Resorcin
Medi-Quik (Sterling)	Spray	Lidocaine	X	Benzalkonium chloride	X
Nupercainal (Ciba)	a. Cream b. Oint. c. Spray	Dibucaine: a. .5% b. 1% c. .25%	X	X	X
Poison Ivy Cream (McKesson)	Cream	Benzocaine	Pyrilamine maleate	Povidone	Zirconium oxide
Pyribenzamine (Ciba)	Cream Oint.	X	Tripelennamine	X	X
Resinol (Resinol)	Oint.	X	X	X	Calamine; Resorcin; Zinc oxide
Surfadil (Lilly)	Oint. Liq.	Cyclomethy-caine	Methapyrilene hydrochloride	X	X
Ziradryl (Parke-Davis)	Liq.	X	Diphen-hydramine; Camphor	X	Zinc oxide

1. An antipruritic relieves itch (pruritus).

7
OTHER DISORDERS

Menstruation and Vaginitis

GENERAL CONSIDERATIONS

Menstruation

Women between the ages of 11 and 55 normally produce a gamete (egg or reproductive cell) according to a regular 28–35 day cycle. If an egg cell is not fertilized, it is expelled through the vagina along with uterine tissue, mucus, and blood. This flow is called menstruation (menses) and typically lasts from 4 to 7 days.

Because the process of egg production involves many organs of your body (brain, bloodstream, ovaries, uterus, etc.), each monthly cycle may have profound and extensive effects on you. Discomfort is usually at its peak prior to and during menstruation. Headache, abdominal cramping, nausea, irritability, swelling (edema), and mild anemia are common.

Non-prescription medications can assist in relieving temporary symptoms of normal menstruation. The use of aspirin or an aspirin substitute can ease headache and the pain of cramping. Diuretics may reduce the discomfort of water retention and swelling. Antihistamines may help relieve nervousness and irritability. Use such medications only for the treatment of regularly recurrent and mild to moderate symptoms. Any profound change in your menstrual cycle requires a doctor's attention.

Vaginitis

At least 20% of American women experience occasional vaginal discomfort unrelated to normal menses. Symptoms include itch, burning, irritation, unpleasant odor, and/or the discharge of bloody mucus. Most symptoms result from imbalances in the vagina caused by hot weather, tight clothing, damp bathing suits, the use of deodorant perfumes, improper vaginal hygiene, and/or excessive douching. Chronic disease such as diabetes, hypertension, or allergies and the use of IUDs or diaphragms may lead to infection or irritation.

Among the more common micro-organisms that may cause infection are a fungus (*Candida albicans*), a bacterium (*Haemophilus vaginalis*), and a protozoan (*Trichomonas vaginalis*). Symptoms include unpleasant odors, episodes of itching and/or pain, and the production of a thick discharge which may be white, gray, or green in color. Such symptoms require your gynecologist's attention.

Good hygiene decreases the possibility of irritation or infection. The frequent replacement of sanitary napkins or tampons is wise. Daily cleansing of the vaginal area with soap and water followed by thorough drying, avoiding vaginal perfumes, minimizing the consumption of sugar, limiting the intake of antibiotics, and immediately changing clothes after swimming are important. If you must douche, avoid the use of irritant sprays, soaps, and powders. Keep your douching equipment clean, do not use bulb syringes, and flush with nothing besides lukewarm water, to which a tablespoon of vinegar may be added.

SELF-TREATMENT

Self-Treatment with a Non-Prescription Menstrual Product May Be Reasonable if—

- your symptoms include mild to moderate headache, nausea, cramping, backache, water retention (edema), irritability, and/or nervous tension.
- your menstrual cycle is regular and your symptoms tend to be repeated with each cycle.
- you are not suffering from any chronic disease.
- you maintain normal but not excessive vaginal hygiene.

Self-Treatment with a Non-Prescription Menstrual Product Is Probably Not Advisable if—

- you have just begun to menstruate or are beginning menopause.
- your normal menstrual cycle is disrupted. Although pregnancy is the most frequent cause of interruption, emotional factors or serious disease conditions may be responsible.

- your symptoms are abnormal, e.g., acute pain, nausea, or non-menstrual vaginal flow.
- you have not had a routine gynecological examination within the past 6 months.
- your symptoms include spasmodic abdominal cramping or persistent aching in the lower abdomen.
- ordinary menstrual flow or the length of menstruation is reduced.
- "spotting" occurs between normal menstrual cycles.
- you have reason to believe that you may have contracted a venereal disease.

Embarrassment concerning menstrual abnormalities often keeps women from seeking essential medical advice. Such fastidiousness can have serious consequences. Any menstrual abnormality requires consultation with your gynecologist or general practitioner.

Before Beginning Self-Treatment with Menstrual Products, It Is Wise—

- to consider whether you have been following intelligent hygienic practices. Regular douching (more than twice a week) can seriously alter the normal vaginal environment. Forgetting to remove tampons or sanitary napkins can create conditions producing irritation, odor, or infection. Perfumes and other cosmetic preparations may cause similar symptoms.
- to consider whether your symptoms may result from abnormal emotional stress or pressure.
- to consider whether you need a routine gynecological examination.
- to consider the other possible conditions which may produce abnormality and discomfort (menopause, pregnancy, psychological factors, chronic disease, or venereal infection).

Ingredients Included in Non-Prescription Medications

Analgesics Aspirin and aspirin substitutes (acetaminophen, salicylates, salicylamides, and phenacetin) are included in many products to reduce the headache or muscular pain often associated with menstruation. A complete discussion of their effectiveness, recommended dosage strength, possible side effects, and adverse reactions is included in Chapter 1. Review those considerations before using any single ingredient or combination product.

Diuretics The retention of water often leads to the swelling (edema) of ankles, legs, and abdomen. Weight gain is generally not large but may aggravate the psychological discomfort and sense of depression which often accompany menstruation. Because such symptoms are temporary, they are best overlooked. However, if a bloated feeling is intolerable, the use of products containing ammonium chloride, caffeine, or pamabrom may help rid you of excessive fluids. Coffee, tea, or cola drinks may have the same diuretic effect.

Antihistamines Phenindamine tartrate, pyrilamine maleate, and methapyrilene fumarate are agents used for treating allergies. They are added to non-prescription sedatives and menstrual products because of their tendency to produce drowsiness. Their sleep-inducing qualities are of questionable advantage in reducing nervousness, irritability, and/or insomnia, particularly during waking hours. Achieving tranquilizing or sedative effects is highly unlikely at the concentrations found in most non-prescription medications.

Mineral Supplements Because of the blood loss associated with menstruation, the possibility of mild anemia has been exploited as a reason for taking dietary supplements containing iron. Any well-balanced diet more than compensates for the loss of this essential mineral.

Other Ingredients The inclusion of such anticholinergics as homatropine or antispasmodics such as cinnamedrine may be medically rational if mucus flow or cramping is excessive. However, concentrations found in non-prescription medications are generally too low to be effective, and the problems they may relieve are better diagnosed and treated by a gynecologist.

PRODUCT CHART

A Selected List of Medications for Menstrual Discomfort

Brand (Manufacturer)	Delivery Form	Analgesic[1]	Antihistamine[2]	Diuretic	Other Active Ingredients[3]
Aqua-Ban (Thompson)	Tab.	X	X	Ammonium chloride, 325 mg; Caffeine, 10 mg	X
Femicin (Norcliff-Thayer)	Tab.	Acetaminophen, 160 mg; Salicylamide, 225 mg	Pyrilamine, 15 mg	X	Homatropine methylbromide, .5 mg (AC)
Humphrey's No. 11 (Hymphrey's)	Tab.	X	X	X	Cimicifuga; Pulsatilla; Sepia
Lydia Pinkham (Smith, Miller & Patch)	Tab.	X	X	X	Extracts: Jamaica dogwood, Pleurisy root, & Licorice; Ferrous (iron) sulfate
Midol (Glenbrook)	Tab.	Aspirin, 454 mg	X	Caffeine, 32 mg	Cinnamedrine, 15 mg (AS)
Pamprin (Chattem)	Tab.	Phenacetin, 125 mg; Salicylamide, 250 mg	Pyrilamine, 12.5 mg	Pamabrom, 25 mg	X
Pre-Mens Forte (Blair)	Tab.	X	X	Ammonium chloride, 500 mg; Caffeine, 100 mg	X
Sunril (Emko)	Cap.	Acetaminophen, 300 mg	Pyrilamine, 25 mg	Pamabrom, 50 mg	X

1. See Chapter 1 for a discussion of medically active analgesics.
2. See Chapter 2 for a discussion of medically active antihistamines.
3. Anticholinergics (AC); Antispasmodics (AS)

Ear, Eye, and Mouth

Ear (Otic) Conditions

You are wise to avoid self-treatment of ear disorders. Accurate diagnosis of conditions producing such typical symptoms as earache, pain, pressure, or oozing requires the professional skills of your doctor or dentist. Infections of the teeth, tongue, jaws, throat, and/or sinuses often cause earache symptoms. Disease conditions arising within the ear itself are usually too serious to be affected by non-prescription medications.

Eye (Ophthalmic) Conditions

The self-treatment of eye disorders is probably not reasonable no matter how trivial your symptoms appear to be. Although simple itching, stinging, tearing, or redness may indicate a minor condition, these same symptoms may be signs of more severe disorders. Self-medication may hide or worsen disease conditions. Consultation with your ophthalmologist is wise, particularly if you have pain or blurred vision. Non-prescription preparations may be all that is needed to treat your condition, but leave that decision to your doctor. This is also true if you wear contact lenses. The advisability and choice of cleaning solutions, artificial tears, decongestants, conditioners, soaking compounds, etc., is best left to the professional who prescribed and fitted your lenses.

Dental Conditions

Methods of caring for your teeth and gums should be determined by your dentist, orthodontist, or periodontist. His or her recommendations will include non-prescription products (waxed or unwaxed dental floss; normal, fluoridated, or anesthetic toothpaste; various forms of mouthwashes; plaque revealer; and/or different types of toothbrush). Wisdom dictates your adherence to these recommendations. The same is true for denture wearers. Professional advice should be sought with the appearance of any pain, discomfort, or chafing. Oral ulcerations (cold or canker sores) are caused by viral infection. Fortunately, they are self-limiting, since no non-prescription drug on the American market is effective in preventing or curing them.[1] Relief from pain or irritation is possible if you use a local anesthetic, but many doctors discourage the use of such medication since it may interfere with the healing process.

---

1. Recent evidence indicates that injections of adenylic acid (available by prescription only) may be helpful.

INDEX

Compounded Undecylenic Acid, 102
Compound W, 105
Compoz, 52
Congespirin, 17
Contac, 39
Coricidin "D", 40
Coricidin Demilets, 40
Coricidin Medilets, 40
Correctol, 70
Coryban-D, 40, 43, 45
Co-Tylenol Cold Formula, 40
Creamalin, 60
Creomulsion, 43
Cuticura, 98

Datril, 22
Deka Expectorant, 43
Delcid, 60
Derma-Soft Creme, 105
Desenex, 102
Desitin, 109
Dex-A-Diet, 93
Dexatrim, 93
Dialose, 70
Dialose Plus, 71
DIA-Quel, 80
Dicarbosil, 60
Diet-Aid, 93
Di-Gel, 60
Dilone, 52
Diothane, 86
Dolor, 18
Dondril Anticough, 43
Donnagel, 80
Donnagel-PG, 80
Dorbane, 71
Dorbantyl, 71
Dorbantyl Forte, 71
Double-E, 53
Doxan, 71
Doxidan, 71
Doxinate, 71
Dramamine, 89
Dr. Caldwell's Senna Laxative, 71
Dr. Scholl's, 105
Dr. Scholl's Corn/Callus, 105
Dristan, 40, 43, 45
Dularin Syrup, 22
Dulcolax, 71

Duradyne, 18
Duragesic, 18

Effersyllium, 71
Elixir Terpin Hydrate, 43
Emetrol, 89
Empirin Compound, 18
Eno, 60
Excedrin, 18
Excedrin P.M., 20, 52
Ex-Lax, 71
Exzit, 98
Exzit Creme/Lotion, 98

Febrinol, 22
Feen-a-Mint, 72
Femicin, 124
Fizrin, 17, 60
Fleet Enema, 72
Fleet Pediatric Enema, 72
Fletcher's Castoria, 72
Foille, 109
Foot-Guard, 102
Fostex, 98
Fostril, 98
Freezone, 105
Fungacetin, 102
Fungi-Spray, 102

Gelusil, 60
Gelusil Flavor Pak, 60
Gelusil-Lac, 60
Gelusil-M, 61
Gentlax, 72
Gentz Wipes, 86
Goody's Headache Powder, 20
Grapefruit Diet Plan with Diadex, 93

Haley's M-O, 61, 72
Hemor-Rid, 86
Hemorr-Aid, see Vaseline Hemorr-Aid
Hista-Calma, 119
Humphrey's No. 11, 124
Hydrolose, 72

Ivy Dry Cream, 119

Kalpec, 80
Kao-Gest, 80
Kaomagma, 80

Kaopectate, 80
Kolantyl, 61
Komed, 99
Krem, 61
Kudrox, 61

Lactinex, 81
Lanacane, 86, 115, 119
Liquiprin, 22
Listerine, 40
Listerine Big 4, 42
Lydia Pinkham, 124

Maalox, 61
Maalox No. 1 & No. 2, 61
Maltsupex, 72
Mamol, 86
Manzan, 87
Maranox, 20
Measurin, 17
Medache, 20
Medi-Quik, 119
Melozets, 93
Mentholatum, 45
Metamucil, 72, 93
Microsyn, 99
Midol, 124
Milk of Magnesia, see Phillips' Milk of Magnesia
Mosco, 105
Mucilose, 73
Mylanta, 61
Mylanta II, 61

Nature's Diet Plan with Diadex, 93
Nature's Remedy, 73
Nebs, 22
Neo-Polycin, 109
Neo-Synephrine, 45
Neo-Synephrine Compound, 40
Neo-Synephrine, Elixir, 41
Nervine, 52
Neutrogena, 99
Nilain, 20
No-Doz, 53
Norwich Elixir, 43
Novahistine DH, 43
Novahistine Expectorant, 43

127